CHAKRA AND REIKI HEALING

A BEGINNERS GUIDE TO LEARN REIKI MEDITATION, DISCOVER THE POWER OF KUNDALINI AND HEAL YOUR CHAKRAS TO INCREASE POSITIVE ENERGY WITH SECRETS OF THIRD EYE AWAKENING

AURORA COOPER

ISBN: 9798635332061

Contents

Introduction 3

Chapter 1. What's Reiki?..6

Chapter 2. The Benefit of Reiki 15

Chapter 3. Reiki Healing Techniques 25

Chapter 4. Reiki Level 36

Chapter 5. Healing Ailments 45

Chapter 6. The Five Reiki Principles 61

Chapter 7. Reiki and Crystals 69

Chapter 8. Reiki And Body Energy 74

Chapter 9. Attunements 81

Chapter 10. Colors of Chakra.................................. 87

Chapter 11. Kundalini Awakening............................. 96

Chapter 12. How To Awaken The Kundalini 101

Chapter 13. Tips For Daily Practice 112

Chapter 14. Conclusion Regarding Reiki 120

Chapter 15. Introduction to Chakras 124

Chapter 16. Identifying Chakras............................ 127

Chapter 17. Chakra Meditation............................. 140

Chapter 18. Healing Your Chakras 151

Chapter 19. The Third Eye And Your Psychic Awakening . 163

Chapter 20. The Ways To Protect Yourself During Third Eye Activation 172

Chapter 21. The Effect Of Yoga On Chakras 183

Chapter 22. Foods That Help With Healing 193

Chapter 23. 7 Signs That Your Chakras Are Out of Balance.. 201

Chapter 24. Chakras, Endocrine System And The Immune System 211

Chapter 25. The Science Behind Chakras................. 221

Chapter 26. Things to Avoid 231

Chapter 27. Conclusion................................... 238

Introduction

The traces of Reiki go far back in human history. In every culture of the world, there were people who had access to higher states of consciousness, and thus timeless wisdom, which they transmitted to humankind and were then passed on, usually orally, by priests, saints, and teachers. There are many indications that in all advanced civilizations - among the Mayans as well as the Egyptians and the ancient Greeks - it was known how to directly tap light energy. In any case, the cosmic symbols on which the Reiki system is based can be found in the Mayan pyramids as well as in the Temple of Luxor.

The historian and Reiki teacher Dr. Barbara Ray traced the roots of Reiki to about 6000 years before Christ and found that they are in northern India and Tibet. The cosmic symbols on which the Reiki system is based are as well known to the Tibetan Lamas as the associated attunement processes.

Dr. Although Mikao Usui (1865-1926) is regarded as the founder of Reiki, but he has not invented this method, but merely rediscovered her and given her the name Reiki. Usui was one of the people who, like many people today, yearned for truth and enlightenment. According to tradition, he lived as the head of a Christian seminary in

Kyoto, Japan, where he was repeatedly asked by his disciples about the phenomenon of the healings that Jesus Christ had accomplished. He knew that Jesus had healed people by laying on hands - that's what the Bible says - but he wondered how that worked. He even traveled to the United States and earned a doctorate in theology from the University of Chicago, but he wasn't any closer to the mystery of the early Christian healings.

Disappointed Usui returned to Japan, learned Sanskrit and began to occupy himself in a monastery with ancient Buddhist scriptures. Finally, he found the key to very ancient knowledge: a Sanskrit formula based on a set of cosmic or universal symbols. Whenever these symbols are activated, they activate the connection to the universal life force. The psychologist Carl Gustav Jung, who has studied cosmic symbols intensively, calls these symbols "foundations of humanity" and "the deepest knowledge available to humanity."

Based on these cosmic symbols is the attunement ritual of Reiki teachers. It goes back to instructions that Usui, according to legend, received in the following ways: He fasted and meditated for 21 days on a sacred mountain near Kyoto. On the last day, he had a light show shortly before sunrise. In front of a wall of light the Sanskrit formula with which he had worked so intensely appeared in golden letters. He took the cosmic symbols on which the entire Reiki system is based, in a certain order true, together with the corresponding attunement processes. All this burned deep into his memory. This experience could be called an experience of enlightenment or cosmic initiation.

According to legend, Usui injured on the way back to the

village on a stone. His toe was bleeding, but when he held his hands over it, the bleeding stopped immediately. Arriving in the valley, he ordered a big Japanese breakfast in an inn. It tasted great, and he tolerated it, even though he had fasted for three weeks. The daughter of the host, who suffered from toothache for days, he laid his hands on briefly - and she was freed from her complaints. These first "healing miracles" exemplify how Reiki can be used: as emergency aid at the scene of an accident, to harmonize bodily functions and in case of both acute and chronic physical and emotional complaints.

Dr. Usui called his method Reiki. Rei means "universal" and Ki means "life force". Reiki means "method for activating universal life force". Initially, Dr. Usui also had many beggars in the slums of Kioto and joined them in Reiki. However, he soon realized that they did not practice it. They preferred the poor but comfortable life of a beggar and did not want to take responsibility for their own lives.

It is also said that Dr. Usui lit a torch in broad daylight in Kyoto and walked up and down the promenade. Asked what he wanted with the torch in bright sunshine, he replied that he was looking for people who wanted to see the true light. This began his lecture and seminar time. At the end of his life, he had taught many people in Reiki and shared his inner knowledge with several advanced disciples. One of these students was Dr. Chujiro Hayashi, who led a private Reiki clinic in Tokyo until 1940.

Chapter 1.
What's Reiki?

What is Reiki? Basic Facts You Should Know

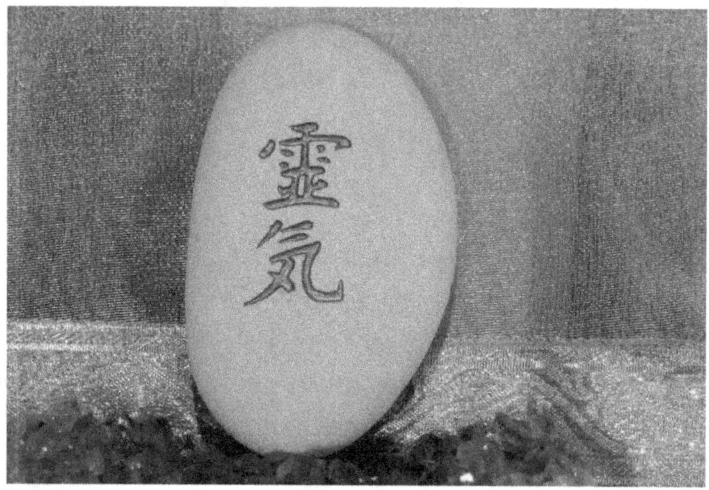

Reiki is a treatment which is popularly known as hands healing in which a professional puts hands softly on or over a patient's body to encourage the patient's process of recuperating.

The word 'Reiki' is a combination of Japanese and Chinese word-characters.

- Rei -- Profound or Powerful

- Ki – imperative vitality

The basic idea shared by the individuals who practice Reiki is that this indispensable vitality can be directed to help the body's natural capacity to mend itself, as indicated by the National Center for Complementary and Integrative Health (NCCIH).

As indicated by these specialists, energy will be low in the body where there has been physical damage or conceivably emotional instability. Sickness itself is a result of these energy reductions.

Energy healing is centered at progressing the flow of vitality and eliminate blocks; this is also done in acupuncture and acupressure. Researchers believe that improving the progression of vitality around the body, can empower unwinding, stop pains, fast recovery, and decrease different manifestations of ailment.

Reiki has been around for a huge number of years. The practice was first created in 1922 by a Japanese Buddhist called Mikao Usui, who purportedly showed 2,000 individuals the Reiki strategy during his lifetime. The training spread to the U.S. through Hawaii during the 1940's, and after that to Europe during the 1980's.

Nonetheless, there is no logical proof to help asserts that alleged fundamental energy really exists, nor is there definitive proof that Reiki is valuable for any wellbeing related purpose, as indicated by the NCCIH. Be that as it may, even though Reiki hasn't been certified as a viable medical tool, that doesn't mean it's a hurtful practice.

According to Ann Baldwin, a teacher of physiology at the University of Arizona and a Reiki expert, Reiki can "do no harm," at worst, the practice can do nothing.

As of late, Reiki has been coordinated into numerous social insurance settings, including medical clinics,

Baldwin disclosed to Live Science. Also, other scientific studies on the practice proposed that this integral treatment might be important for diminishing tension and torment, relaxing, improving exhaustion and mitigating the side effects of depression, indicating by the Center for Spirituality and Healing at the University of Minnesota (UMN).

Essential Things you MUST Remember Before Reiki

Some Reiki experts and novice tend to forget some things when practicing Reiki. You must be aware of these few basic knowledges that is identified with the act of self-treatment and medications accomplished for other people. With this knowledge, you are better informed about the practice

Reiki Heals What Must Be Healed

The healing is not based on what we want to heal. A few people say that "Reiki is an astute vitality" and that it flows where the recuperating will really occur. The truth is, Reiki is not all about insight, but about its distinctive capacity to restore healing in a place where it was lost. This is overlooked here and there, individuals attempt to force the process, and they feel terrible when Reiki didn't give the results they were seeking after. Actually, this happens to every first timer – including me.

Reiki will only flow and heal, bringing in harmony the things that must be healed, in a way they can be really get healed – nothing else will occur. Each Reiki expert is only a channel for the vitality and has restricted command over this Reiki power.

Make sure to mend the origin of the problem, and not the

manifestations: this is the right expectation and it should be the mindset when you are practicing Reiki. For instance, you may experience an individual with a migraine and do Reiki to bring relief from discomfort. Yet even with the good intention of your heart, the aim must be somewhat unique: to recuperate the source of the pain. At the point when the origin is healed, the manifestations are no more existing.

The side effects may not vanish immediately, so keep that in mind and advise this to the individual who approaches you for Reiki. Try not to be disheartened by this and discontinue doing Reiki, note that occasionally, time is fundamental if the origin of the pain is to regain healing.

The Effects of Reiki is Important to Every Customer

By "customer" I mean any individual who approaches you for Reiki: it can be a relative or a companion who is not giving you a dime for it.

At whatever point you offer Reiki to somebody, make certain to disclose to this individual the idea of Reiki healing process. Clarify that first, Reiki mends not the indications, but the root and center of the issue. The side effects may not vanish immediately, so tell the individual to remain patient. Next, make sure you clarify the idea of "purifying" period after Reiki sessions. Most times, this is really the same as what you have encountered after Reiki attunement, or after concentrated self-practice. There are times when the side effects may become more grounded, which is due to the body connected with its self-healing systems.

During the period, synchronicity occurs, and that

customer may see a lot of signs throughout his life, disclosing to him what changes he should grasp, and what things he ought to dispose of from his/her life. If you fail to explain this prior to the session, the person will be afraid to continue Reiki.

Additionally, ensure that the individual desires are healing. A few people simply would prefer not to heal; there are numerous purposes behind that. Check the customer's aim before you start the treatment. If a person believes that healing is not important to him, the exercise might become useless.

The Reiki Precepts are a Central Part of Reiki

The Five Reiki Precepts are frequently disregarded; this is wrong. But then in all actuality, these statutes are basic aspects of Reiki practice and Reiki can't be truly utilized effectively without incorporating these statutes into the life of the expert. They resemble rules, demonstrating to you the ideal approach to healing, by making changes in five extraordinary fields of life – feelings, considerations, appreciation, self-development and empathy to everything in the world. Reiki medications give you the healing energy, yet the rules show you the way. Also, everybody can utilize these statutes. If you are healing others, it is good to tell them about these precepts.

Usui proposed that the statutes ought to be rehashed (ruminated and thought about upon) every day and every morning, best with your hands in a Gassho mudra.

Rehash these statutes thrice toward the beginning of the day and thrice at night, depending on your needs. You can likewise ponder upon the guidelines and thoroughly consider your life as per these standards.

Most experts believe that the two basic ideas behind Reiki are: self-medications and, precisely, the precepts of Reiki. By coordinating the two components into your day by day life, you are on the way to self-healing.

Music Improves the Practice

Background music during Reiki treatment (or self-treatment) is a good thought. It is a good idea because a piece of nice, delicate music improves the conditions of relaxations and quiets the dawn. You would enjoy the use of music when treating yourself or others. With the music, you send the Reiki vitality effectively, and if you are treating others, they get to experience the effect better. Also, background sounds make you achieve better results from each session.

Yet, recall that the music must be delicate and serene. It is anything but wise to play Heavy Metal. Find out which sounds are most suitable for Reiki sessions. Also, find out which music makes you relaxed normally; this includes the music preference of the person you want to heal.

Additionally, keep in mind that the deeper the relaxation, the deeper your hearing. Therefore, as the exercise progresses, the music might become so loud than when you started; and this can be annoying. Therefore, ensure that the music is calm enough; the ideal approach to do so is to play the music, loosen up for 30 minutes and see what volume works best.

However, you should use legal music to avoid any unfavorable situations. There are sites with free sounds that you can get legally.

Be Cautious About Incenses and Fragrance Oils

Numerous professionals appreciate utilizing incenses or scent oils during Reiki treatment. They give this decent, healing and mystical state of mind. Yet, before picking up just any fragrance, you must keep some things in mind.

To begin with, a few out of every odd individual prefer incenses or oils. Furthermore, regardless of whether the individual like these, it doesn't mean the person in question likes that particular aroma and type you wish to utilize. For instance, there are two kinds of scent oils – characteristic (and costly) and fake (typically toxic). It is advisable to use normal oils.

For incenses, there are two sorts of these too – regular and costly, and fake and poisonous. What's more, there are numerous sorts of these incenses with regards to shape and fixings. Incense sticks with wood powder, stick on a bamboo, cones, pitches or incense powders, all of which performs distinctively.

In all honesty, the ideal approach to buy incenses is to look for them on Etsy, where many individuals handcraft these. Inquire as to whether the incense is 100% organic, which is what you should use. The natural White Sage or herbs like this can be utilized as incenses, as well.

Try not to use cheap and poisonous incenses that are regularly sold in profound stores. High-quality incenses are great, however once a major organization begins to make incenses, the impact of their work is normally upsetting.

Ensure That Your Client Is Comfortable

You can't disregard your customer's solace. Keep in mind

that when an individual rests on a bed, his temperature may appear lower due to the slow progression of the blood. In simpler terms, the person you are healing might get cold since he is not moving. Ensure you have prepared a cover for the individual when this occurs.

Also, the proper position on the bed is important for comfort. If you do Reiki sessions on a regular schedule, it's best to get yourself a back-rub table. Put a pad under your head or the person's, for one. Likewise, place a pad or something comparative under the knees, as it will loosen up this locale of the body, as well. Lastly, place a cushion or something comparative under the lower legs – once more, this will enable the body to unwind.

Remember About Self-Treatment

Self-treatment is the most well-known approach to work with Reiki, yet you can likewise learn Japanese systems of contemplation (for instance, from the prescribed The Reiki Sourcebook) and utilize these. There are numerous strategies to look over, for example, Gassho reflection, Joshin Kokyu Ho and so on.

Recuperating and developing yourself is the fundamental component of Reiki practice – which, from multiple points of view, is simply the way improvement and self-mending. Attempt to work with Reiki vitality for at any rate 30 minutes out of every day. Also, remember that sending Reiki to your nourishment or plants is additionally an approach to rehearse.

You're not a Doctor – Don't Play One

In case you're not a specialist of medication, don't diagnose or prescribe anything to people. Try not to propose explicit medicinal issues to your patients. In the event that you see something dangerous that you don't care for (in light of the fact that you've read a couple of restorative books), don't call it, don't discuss it, simply recommend the customer to proceed to visit an expert therapeutic authority.

Frequently, your customer may ask "you touched my liver – do I have liver issues?!" in such or comparable cases, you can just say that you do Reiki dependent on instinct and what you feel where you ought to send Reiki and you don't generally have a clue why you ought to do this with the exception of the way that you feel this is correct. Possibly, you ought to disclose to the customer the strategy of Byosen Reikan Ho.

Try not to Commercialize Practice Too Much

The act of Reiki is intended to heal your own life. However, you should not learn it for the sole purpose of becoming a Reiki expert or educator. Actually, it is not really a good idea to be a Reiki instructor because you might lose your healing while trying to heal others (most especially beginners that do not entirely want to be healed)

Frequently, Reiki will demonstrate to you your actual gifts that have nothing to do with healing. Understand that while it is natural for some people to become Reiki experts, others will continue to struggle with it. Nevertheless, keep in mind that Reiki has a lot to do with healing rather than making money.

Chapter 2.
The Benefit of Reiki

Reiki has many benefits, including healing the body, mind, and spirit but it also helps promote balance and harmony both within the body and our environment. Reiki is a non-invasive healing energy that helps enhance and promote the body's natural healing abilities while encouraging the flow of Ki which overall enhances the body's wellbeing. Reiki can restore balance on all levels within the body and it can directly heal the problem instead of just taking away the pain or relieving some symptoms.

In terms of balance, Reiki can create an emotional and mental balance between the good and the bad. When healing the body from its problem, you are putting less stress on the mind, which affects the mental and emotional state of the human brain. Balance comes from when a person is able to live free from any worries about their own bodies. When there is no stress, there is no anger meaning many negative feelings simply fade away, leaving the body with a balanced and harmonized mindset. Reiki has also the power to heal depression, anxiety, negative emotions, and many other mental illnesses.

Reiki can also relieve any tension within the body and stress itself. When the treatment is in process, Reiki doesn't just go through a particular part of the body that has a problem, it might start with that part, but it makes itself flow all throughout the body, relaxing it and releasing of any stress and tension. Many practitioners reported feeling relaxed, clear-minded, lighter, and peaceful after performing Reiki on themselves or after Reiki has been done on them. This is because the energy flows everywhere, releasing tension that has been put on any parts within your body.

Many of today's known diseases are linked to a stress factor such as work stress, environmental stress, or even emotional stress. This leads to irregular heart rhythms that can cause a stroke, angina, gastrointestinal problems, eating disorders, mood disorders, sexual problems, and many psychological problems. Reiki can help you regulate this stress to avoid any problems within the mind and body.

You are able to achieve natural balance with the body, mind, and spirit due to Reiki dissolving any chakra or energy blocks. These energy blocks can also affect the body physically or mentally. When Reiki is done regularly, it can bring a more peaceful and calmer state to the body and person who is dealing with stress in their everyday lives. The mental balance can also enhance mental clarity, memory, and learning, as well as heal emotional or mental wounds, frustrations, anger, mood swings, fear, and even personal relationships. In general, Reiki enhances your ability to give love and receive love, making you more open to any people and relationships around you.

Reiki is able to give one space where they are able to become more aware of what is happening within their bodies, causing them to make decisions that change the way they live their lives in terms of diet, habits, etc. Many practitioners even report changing their habits or abandoning them. When you become more present of what is happening within your body, you start to access inner wisdom or knowledge. It changes your point of view on certain things in your environment or life.

We are so easily affected by the stress we experience every day in our lives that sometimes it even becomes our 'normal,' and our bodies completely forget what it's like to be in balance once again. Many practitioners can tell you that Reiki is a wonderful and gentle healing practice that makes their body and mind feel amazing, that is the body's true, normal, and balanced nature. It can be rather difficult to maintain this balance but that is why Reiki can be practiced regularly to ensure the body is able to return to its balanced state. Reiki is able to remind our body how to shift into its own self-healing mode even when Reiki is not being practiced. This parasympathetic nervous system state allows you to digest and sleep better, which is very important when it comes to the body's health and vitality. The more often you are able to achieve this state, the more you can become productive and active without the feelings of exhaustion, stress, or burnout floating inside you.

Reiki improves your connection to the Universe and nature. It also has the power to ground and center you by improving focus within the mind. With the help of this energy and your mind, you will be able to stay centered in this present moment instead of living in the past and always being stopped by guilt and regrets from moving on and living your best life. Reiki can help strengthen the ability that revolves around accepting yourself and any events that happen around you, even if they are not aligned with your desires or goals. Instead of acting out of habit, you are able to be more supportive of yourself and others around you; Reiki can help you look at the brighter things when life throws you challenges.

As mentioned above, Reiki can promote better relaxation, which aids in better sleep. With sleep and relaxed bodies, the healing process can go by more smoothly and at a faster rate. You are also able to think more clearly, become focused, and move forward on your spiritual path. This deep relaxation releases many tensions within the body, making it finally function smoothly which is different from your old toxic and tense body. Many practitioners who practice Reiki on themselves or during their attunement, report falling into a deep sleep due to the deep relaxation they experience.

After Reiki has been performed, your body goes to your natural state, accelerating the self-healing ability drastically. During this period, your heart rate, blood pressure, and breathing improve. You will be able to inhale and exhale more deeply and easier than before, this is usually one of the first things that show improvement after performing Reiki on yourself or when someone does Reiki on you. Deep breathing naturally settles our minds, and oxygen also helps fight cancer!

A Reiki treatment is able to restore balance on a very deep level, encouraging the system to improve the body's vital functions such as sleeping, breathing, and digesting. On a more physical level, Reiki is able to relieve the pain and symptoms of sciatica, migraines, arthritis, asthma, menopausal symptoms, chronic fatigue, insomnia, and many other illnesses. Reiki can also help stimulate and increase mobility in many cases of lower back pain, wrist pain, and shoulder pain. It also has the power to heal inflammations and infections within the body. Reiki, done on yourself or sent to someone over distance healing, has proven to work efficiently as told by many of those who received Reiki and perform Reiki on others. It can also improve indices of the metabolic syndrome which is associated with a risk of type two diabetes, many chronic conditions, and even heart disease.

Not only does Reiki cleanse the body physically, but spiritually too. Cleansing both the mind and body helps promote spiritual growth and personal development. Although you do not need to be spiritual to receive Reiki, it does help in your spiritual path. Instead of targeting individual symptoms, Reiki goes through the entire body. Often a practitioner receives messages, change of attitude, visions, or see things from a different point of view. It makes you see your condition in a new light and makes you deal with it in another and more positive way.

When one is relaxed, the healing process is accelerated. Reiki is a very gentle treatment that can be used on medical conditions such as diabetes, heart conditions, epilepsy, and many others. Reiki also supports chemotherapy. Reiki can also support women on any stage during their pregnancy and gives them the energy to carry on their day-to-day activities.

Many people often replace therapy with a Reiki practice, which is able to give you more self-love, enable you to connect with people on a more emotional level, strengthen your relationships, and solve problems that occur outside of your body. The way we think and what intentions we set for ourselves affect the environment around us; for example, when someone is always angry, their environment will be full of negative energy which can attract many problems and disappointment instead of desires and goals. Having clean thoughts and mindset can help you achieve your goals, Reiki can do that and so much more!

Reiki heals very fast, sometimes even way too quickly. Especially when it comes to healing emotional traumas or mental disorders, there are always negative feelings that occupy our thoughts. Many people go through something called the 'healing crisis,' which is a phase of the body in which the self-healing process started to work by vanishing any negativity and stress out of the system. In order for anyone to move on from something that is bothering them, either mentally or physically, one must first accept and acknowledge the situation. This is what happens in the 'healing crisis,' the energy acknowledges what the issue is and started to remove it from your system. Sometimes this healing process works way too fast, releasing emotions that you've been holding on for quite some time in order to heal yourself on a deeper level.

It's the same concept as fevers. When the body senses a virus from the outside of the body, it raises the temperature drastically, giving one fever and killing that virus in the process. The body just releases all that energy and emotions all at once, and for those who suffered very painful past traumas, it can be a very poor experience having all those emotions back up and running through your head. Many practitioners or clients report crying or yelling a lot during this time, but one shouldn't let these emotions get the better of them. It's simply the final step to releasing the negativity and moving on. Don't get too attached to that moment in your past but think of it as a challenge in life that you have overcome.

It is also not recommended to use Reiki for healing broken bones. Since Reiki is fast healing energy, broken bones might heal the wrong way and will require breaking them again for them to heal in the right direction. Reiki is a pure form of healing energy unless the practitioner or Reiki master uses the energy in the wrong way; there are no serious side effects.

On a more mental level, Reiki can help reduce anxiety and depression by changing your mood. When you feel more relaxed and less stressed, you feel more calm and happy about yourself and your environment, but when you are angry, you often take this feeling out on yourself and others around you. Changes in mood are associated with depression and anxiety. Many studies have proven that there is an overall improvement to one's mood after Reiki, these improvements lead to a reduction of confusion, fear, doubt, depression, anger, and anxiety in many practitioners. Loss of vigor, which is one of the symptoms of depression, returns to its original state once depression dissolves, which then improves the body's mental state.

Overcoming anxiety and reducing negative thoughts is the goal of a healthy body. A research study published in 2006 had a goal determining if Reiki can actually reduce anxiety in women who were experiencing hysterectomies. Those who received the Reiki treatments experienced having a drastic reduction in anxiety than those who were in the control groups. This study, however, only applied to women who were undergoing surgery. Another research carried in Turkey wanted to determine whether Reiki treatment can reduce pain, fatigue, and anxiety among cancer patients. The study found that those who had a Reiki treatment done on them had experienced a reduction and improvement in all these variables. Another different study aimed to discover where treating older adults would improve their anxiety, depression, and some other issues. Yet again, the results didn't disappoint. Many participants of that study reported that not only did their symptoms fade away, but they experienced complete relaxation during a Reiki treatment.

It is safe to say that you, too, can heal your anxiety and many other issues with the help of Universal life energy. But first things first, you must learn a bit more about this amazing and pure energy before jumping into the healing process. Reiki isn't just done on oneself but it can be performed on others too, such as people, animals, events, and plants.

Self-healing is the most popular practice. There are many different ways and techniques of one performing Reiki on themselves. This works by using your hands and placing them in a certain position above countless parts of your body, from top to bottom to ensure that the energy travels everywhere.

Hands-on-healing is the most basic form of healing that revolves around giving the healing energy to someone who is physically present with you. You ask the person to lie down in order for them to relax completely, with their eyes closed and in a comfortable position. The healing begins with the practitioner's hands hovering above the crown chakra and making their way throughout the other chakras in the patient's body.

Distant healing involves a practitioner performing Reiki on another that is not physically present in the moment. When performing distant healing, you must ask the person to have some time to themselves to relax, sit down with their eyes closed and legs crossed for a couple of minutes while you perform the Reiki healing. Reiki can also be done on those who don't believe in the process or those who never had Reiki done on them before. Reiki can also be done to those who are unaware that this process is happening to them. Distant healing energy can also be sent using object forms, such as a photograph or an image of them, an intention slip, or an object that belongs to them.

Distant healing can also be used for occasions or events such as healing broken relationships or sending love and healing to families who are going through tough times. Reiki can be used on past events such as heartbreak or childhood traumas. Reiki doesn't have the power to change the past, but it can help you move on and change the way you feel about that event. Such as changing fear into strength.

Reiki can also be used on other living things such as plants and animals. Applying the same hands-on-healing but slightly changing your intentions can help. For an animal or pet that requires healing, simply focus and hover your hands around the animal. It can be difficult for them to stay still, which is why it is best given when the animal is asleep. For plants, sending Reiki through roots to promote faster and stronger growth, it can also be used on soil, water, seeds.

Reiki helps the body in self-purification, thus promoting immunity. There are much energy and time needed to fight stress and its causes that dictate the nature of lives. At long last, we forget to balance our lives. Our bodies are tuned to the game of stress management naturally until there is no room for relaxation. When Reiki comes in, it acts as a sympathizer that brings us to rest so that we can experience a moment of healing. At this stage, you will still remain active as usual and much productive. The difference will be that your body will be given more room to rest and meditate which is essential for body health and strength. When you allow Reiki in your life, it makes life more productive and active, free from stress and exhaustion or depletion.

Frees Up the Mindset, Makes You More Focused, Rooted, and Stable. You will remain composed and in a steadier condition as opposed to, overthinking over the past events, or even worrying for the future unknowns. Reiki lets you live today as a day and not live in the past or the future. At the end of the day, you will feel sober even when the conditions are not favorable to you, especially in your work environment. Instead of allowing the situations to control you, you will be in a position to challenge them and stand out as strong as if there was no challenge at all. You will end up being of great help to others who feel low or weak as a result of stress or de-motivation.

Chapter 3.
Reiki Healing Techniques

What keeps us alive is the energy of life in our bodies. Energy flows through our bodies and it also flows outside of us. It flows through the physical body along pathways known as chakras. These are also sometimes referred to as meridians or nadis. Lifeforce flows outside us and around our bodies in a space known as the aura. It acts to nourish the cells and organs in our bodies. It supports them to remain functioning at an optimum level. When the energy becomes disrupted, certain organs and tissues within our bodies can diminish.

This energy is directly linked to our beliefs and emotions. Therefore, it can also be disrupted when we entertain bad beliefs or emotions about ourselves. This includes whether these beliefs and emotions are conscious or unconscious. Negative thoughts and emotions get caught in our flow of energy and result in disrupting the energy's flow. This then affects the functions of our bodies.

Reiki helps the body by carrying energy along with the damaged parts of the body. It recharges each part with good energy and gets rid of the negative energy that exists there. It increases our overall vibration levels both in the body and in the aura. This raising of energy levels lowers the effect of the negative thoughts and emotions as they break apart. This allows Reiki to clear and heal the energy blockages, enabling energy to be guided naturally and healthily through the body.

How Reiki Healing Works: The Theory

When looked at from the most obvious level, it is clear that Reiki treatment has a direct impact on lowering stress levels and releasing tension from the system. Further than this, it also helps a person move towards a better balance in body, mind and spirit. Even more, it can help the body's own natural healing mechanisms to kick in again and begin to function more effectively.

What Exactly Is Reiki Doing?

So, the question is, how does Reiki lower stress and help enable the body to heal? An exact answer to this question remains to be found. However, there have been increasing levels of research covering the effects of Reiki. There is now evidence showing its effect on lowering heart rate, blood pressure, and stress hormones. It has also been shown to improve immune strength. While we have evidence to show the effects Reiki has, we can only offer broad theories as to what causes these effects and how exactly the healing is occurring.

Reiki affects us on multiple levels and often with immediate results. This suggests that Reiki is a complex process that interacts with many of the body's systems simultaneously. It results in the body shifting from a stressed state, also known as fight-or-flight mode, to one of relaxation, where the body is primed to heal itself–this is referred to as a parasympathetic state. Many scientists suggest that this shift is triggered on a subconscious level in an area referred to as the biofield.

What Is the Biofield?

The biofield refers to an area that surrounds the physical body. Medical science has adopted the term to explain the vibrational energy field that is believed to exist in this space. There is no way of actually studying the biofield as current technology is not yet capable of verifying its existence. Having said this, traditional and indigenous cultures have recognized this biofield of energy for thousands of years, and it has always been believed to be a cornerstone of health and wellbeing. Any disruption to this biofield was seen as a loss in balance and the beginning of an illness. So, just because science has not developed far enough to examine this phenomenon, it does not mean it should be dismissed. The wisdom from indigenous cultures runs much deeper than science, which is a relatively new faculty in terms of human history.

Many healing traditions from indigenous cultures use vibration to restore the necessary balance to the mind and body. We can see evidence of this in practices such as ceremonial drumming, chanting rituals, and humming. There is plenty of science to support the therapeutic benefits of vibration through music and sounds. This has led musicians to purposely construct music that can raise or lower people's energies to the desired level. One song called Weightless was developed by Marconi Union to help relieve stress. The song is said to decrease stress levels by up to 60% once listened to with closed eyes. You can feel the vibrational shift through listening to the song as your body's natural rhythm realigns itself. Some say that Reiki's healing benefits are derived from a similar vibrational mechanism, one which increases the level of coherence in the body and decreases the level of dissonance.

Another theory suggests that a Reiki practitioner's hands hold the power of the energetic vibrations which are transmitted to the recipient. These vibrations are then passed from the practitioner to the client to induce healing. The effect could then cause the client to have a shift in awareness as they recognize the healing power they hold within is the key to their wellbeing, regardless of their current state of health. Reiki could then be seen as helping a person resync back to health, similar to how grandfather clocks in the same room adjust to the rhythm of the main clock or how we, too, become relaxed in the presence of someone who is very peaceful. Reiki can connect the practitioner with a deep, inner peace regardless of how they are feeling at that moment.

Many other therapies aim to restore the biofield's balance. These include yoga, acupuncture, qigong, and shiatsu to name but a few. Reiki is one of the most subtle of these therapies as it uses mainly vibrations rather than physical manipulation or even gentle force. It is also suggested by some that Reiki does not act in the biofield at all but rather another field known as the unified field. Some believe that Reiki is more similar to meditation than other energy therapies.

Reiki Compared to Other Treatments

According to the NCCIH, Reiki is an alternative medicine practice that complements existing practices by using energy that is still to be measured by science. Most energy healing methods presume that humans inhabit a certain type of energy which both runs through us and around us. It is believed that energy therapies such as Healing Touch help to bring equilibrium to these energies.

As mentioned, many Reiki practitioners see Reiki as completely distinct to most energy healing and more akin to meditative practices. Many energy healing methods use specific ways to gain access to a person's biofield to make alterations; Reiki does not try to diagnose problems or purposely alter the energy field. They are more passive in their involvement as the energy finds its path.

Reiki practice by nature is extremely passive. A practitioner's hand does not move for most of the treatment duration. The only time they do is alter placements of the hands. A Reiki practitioner is a neutral party; they do not make an effort to change a person or change their energy field. A Reiki practitioner does not try to harness and use Reiki energy; they simply rest their hands on a person's body. Sometimes, they will rest their hands just above the body, in cases where there is an open wound or burn that needs to be healed.

The energy that arises in a practitioner's hands comes naturally as it responds to the needs of the individual for balance in certain areas. Because of this, every treatment is tailored to meet the specific needs of that person, although the practitioner often uses a similar process for every session.

Reiki is best administered in a complete session; however, it can also be given in a shorter session to tackle certain points of a person's body. In pressing circumstances, even a few minutes of Reiki makes a big difference.

How Reiki Healing Is Done: The Healing Session

Reiki session has no standard or even a set time limit or exact protocol to be adhered to. It is allowed to be performed by anyone who has received the necessary training. This might be someone who is professionally qualified, but it can also be a healthcare provider or a friend or member of your family; it could even be you. There is also no typical setting required for Reiki. Generally, Reiki works best somewhere quiet, but it can be performed anywhere, regardless of what is going on in the vicinity and no matter what is happening to the person receiving it. A few moments of Reiki often brings relaxation to emergencies. It is often administered directly after injuries occur and even during and after surgeries. We will also cover modified sessions.

Who Should I See?

To give yourself the best experience possible, you must take the time to do some research before choosing a practitioner that you believe you can be comfortable with. You should decide whether you want to receive Reiki from a friend or a professional you do not know. If you have a friend that you feel very comfortable with, it can help improve the bonding experience. However, if you are not naturally comfortable with strangers, you may want to choose a professional for a greater level of experience. Try to meet with your practitioner beforehand to get a feel for the person and to know what to expect from the session.

Look for a practitioner who describes the process to you clearly and details how they plan to structure the session. This will help you know what to expect when going into the session, and it will make you more at ease. Your personal experience of Reiki will be very different from most others, but if you know what to expect before going in, it always helps.

What Is the Setting?

The most beneficial setting is one where it is quiet and where you will not be disturbed. Most professional Reiki practitioners will have a space dedicated to their practice. If they are doing house calls, they will usually have plenty of knowledge of how best to set up an optimal space. Practitioners often play soft music during sessions to promote relaxation through ambient sounds. If you prefer to have no music, however, do not be afraid to let your practitioner know.

The length of sessions can vary widely. For those receiving Reiki in hospitals and nursing homes, sessions tend to only last around twenty minutes. Professional practitioners provide treatments that last up to ninety minutes. Most Reiki treatments are in between the two.

How Do I Sign Up?

Many practitioners will provide clients with intake forms and will conduct a screening interview beforehand to discover the client's health history or if any underlying issues need to be raised. However, because of the nature of Reiki and its origins, many practitioners avoid these types of processes as they are more associated with mainstream medical practices. Reiki is often seen as more informal and less structured than typical medical procedures. Many times, you will need to fill out a consent form.

Next, the entire process will be explained to you and the

practitioner will ask if you have any specific needs or requests. It is your job to inform the practitioner if you suffer from any conditions that may affect the session, especially if lying flat on your back or front will be a problem or if there are any places where you are sensitive to touch. In some more formal places, such as hospitals or healthcare environments, a practitioner may have to ask if they are allowed to use their hands on the body.

What Is Involved in a Session?

A full Reiki session requires the recipient to be lying down or upright in a comfortable chair.

Usually, Reiki is performed with soft touches, where the practitioner's hands are placed in multiple locations. These include the head and front and back of a person's belly area. A practitioner should not put their hands in private places, and they should not feel intrusive.

Extra placements on injured parts of the body may be performed as needed, such as on the arm for a surgical scar. The practitioner can also hold their hands just above the affected area if it is sore to the touch, providing the same treatment benefits.

What Is the Experience Like?

The experience of Reiki is very subjective. Sometimes, the changes are very subtle and not initially noticeable to the recipient. However, there seems to be an array of shared experiences many people feel during a Reiki treatment.

Some people quote a feeling of heat emanating from the practitioner's hands, while others note a refreshingly cool feeling coming from their hands. Some also experience a pulsating effect where the practitioner's hands are placed as waves of energy pulsate and flow through the body.

A lot of people comment on how comforting the experience is. One study reported how recipients regularly felt that they were hovering in an altered state of consciousness while, at the same time, being fully aware of their surroundings and drawn deeply within. Others have reported falling into a deep, meditative state, while some find the experience to be quite dramatic. Some find their first Reiki session to be not very eventful, but they often report feeling good afterward. The usual resulting feeling is one of deep relaxation and an instant release of stress.

Reiki is a compounding practice and even those who do not notice much on their first time, usually get deeper and more profound experiences as they continue their sessions. Aside from the immediate after-effects of Reiki treatment, you may also experience other positive changes in the days afterward. These include better digestion, a more centered feeling as opposed to being reactive, and better and deeper sleep.

What Should I Do During the Session?

Once you have chosen a practitioner that you believe you will feel comfortable with and that has adequate skills and knowledge of Reiki, then there is not much you can do during a session other than to relax and to trust in the practitioner.

If you want to try and improve your Reiki experience however, you can try some of these tips:

Bring some music that you find relaxing to you.

Go to the bathroom before the session so that you can lie down comfortably without the distraction of feeling the need to go to the toilet.

If you are very sensitive to being touched, it might help if you ask the practitioner beforehand what areas they plan to touch so that you know exactly what will happen during the session.

Tell the practitioner of your requirements before the session starts. If you struggle to lay flat or you have difficulty breathing in certain positions, then let them know and they can work on an alternative. Or if you have had surgery recently and are especially sensitive in an area, let them know so they can avoid causing you pain by touching it. Also, if you happen to be pregnant or are suffering from digestive problems, you may not be able to lie on your stomach. Let them know and they can help.

As the session goes on, you should begin to feel more relaxed. If you become uncomfortable, however, be sure to adjust your position. If there is anything else you need to improve your comfort, whether it be a blanket or support for your lower back, make sure to let the practitioner know. This process is designed to help you after all, and the practitioner wants to make sure the experience is as pleasant and comfortable as possible for you.

Do not try to force yourself into relaxation during Reiki. Reiki is a passive experience, and you should naturally be relaxed through the session. Feel free to let your mind wander; listen to the music and your breathing as well as the feelings you experience during the session.

How Does the Session End?

Unlike most other treatments, Reiki does not give a diagnosis, so do not expect one. Practitioners may make some standard recommendations to you such as drink more fluids or to listen to your body.

While most individuals feel refreshed after Reiki, some people note that they feel more tired than usual that evening. This does not mean they reacted badly to the treatment; it is a natural response from the body to be tired after undergoing healing. People often report a rich feeling of calm and clarity after Reiki as well as very good sleep.

What is the Optimum Number of Sessions?

The person you visit might recommend several sessions to you. The traditional number of sessions is four. This tends to give you enough time to evaluate the benefits, if any, you are receiving. You should take the time to discuss how it would be most suitable to arrange the sessions to get the maximum benefits based on your needs and your schedule.

When you are facing a serious illness, most people would suggest a series of four sessions completed in less than one week. They do not necessarily have to be given by the same practitioner.

Chapter 4.
Reiki Level

Many people seek the benefits of the healing practice of Reiki simply as patients suffering from a variety of physical, psychological, emotional, or spiritual ailments. Such patients may only have learned of Reiki after first being diagnosed with their illness. Many patients may feel "stuck" in their lives or dissatisfied with the results of treatment for their medical doctors. By seeking out a practitioner of Reiki, they may hope to find more complete relief from their condition.

Although Reiki healing is not regulated by any governmental agency medical board, or psychological or psychiatric society, the international community of Reiki practitioners continues to follow the basic methods outlined by the founder of Reiki healing practice. Since its founding, the various schools of Reiki healing have developed several variations and methods of both practice and teaching, but all of them conform to a uniform structure. Certification as a Reiki practitioner is awarded in 3 levels—First Degree, Second Degree, and Third Degree, or the Reiki Master level. To be considered qualified to practice Reiki, the practitioner must have attained at least a First Degree certification from a qualified teacher.

First Degree Reiki

First Degree Reiki training is open to anyone who wishes to learn to use Reiki energy healing. There are no prerequisites. The Japanese word for First Degree is Shoden. Basically, First Degree Reiki training includes the study of the official history and tradition of Reiki, an introduction to the use of Reiki for self-treatment as well as for treating others, and an initial attunement that enables the student to begin accessing the powerful force of Reiki energy.

One of the important distinctions of First Degree Reiki training is that it is open to all students and prospective teachers.

A second important characteristic of First Degree Reiki training is its focus on the physical applications of Reiki. However, when students are attuned to Reiki at the First Degree level, the energy they are able to access functions almost exclusively at the physical level. Students who receive attunement in First Degree training will be expected to perform Reiki healing mostly on themselves but will also receive instruction for healing others by transmitting to them the energy that flows through their hands.

Each student will have a unique experience at this level, but typically attunement results in feelings of heat or coolness, or sensations such as tingling or buzzing that occurs in the hands and fingers. Some students have reported feeling an immediate shift in their perceptions with the sense of Reiki flowing through them occurring immediately at the time of attunement. Others have reported a short delay, with sensations beginning a few hours after the intitule attunement. Still others have reported delays of up to a month or more before they notice any change. For this reason, there is usually a required waiting period between First Degree Reiki and Send Degree Reiki training sessions.

The main focus in First Degree Reiki is to help the student learn how to use Reiki on himself or herself. During attunement, the teacher will spend time opening the channels that flow from the crown chakra and opens the student the increased capacity for healing at this level. As a result, there is an expectation that the student will be working toward resolving any issues that may be blocking the passage of energy through the chakras, as well as any other problems or concerns that brought them into Reiki training to begin with.

Once the student is connected to the Universal Energy during the initial attunement, he or she remains connected for the rest of his or her life. The amount and degree of healing energy each student may be able to access after the initial attunement may vary widely from one student to the next, but as the student becomes increasingly proficient and comfortable using the healing energy, the intensity and constancy of this energy tends to grow and then stabilize.

First Degree training represents an abrupt shift in the student's priorities and way of living. In addition, First Degree training includes initial attunement. Because these significant developments require some time to seek their own level, many teachers will require that students practice self-Reiki, continue focusing on opening their energy channels, and ensure they are committed to the healing practice before continuing to the next level.

It is also important to note that early in its development,

First Degree Reiki training was comprised of four discrete levels: Loku-Tou, Go-Tou, Yon-Tou and San-Tou. When Dr. Takata introduced a Westernized model of Reiki to her audience, she combined these four levels into one level, but required that First Degree students undergo four separate attunements. These evolutionary developments in the way in which knowledge of Reiki healing has been communicated around the world may account for any differences you encounter when you pursue Reiki training at this level.

Second Degree Reiki

Second Degree Reiki training is characterized by the initiation of students to the treatment of others. Specifically, Second Degree Reiki training is training at the Practitioner level; successful completion of his level entitles students to begin charging patients for providing healing treatment.

To be accepted into a Second Degree Reiki training class, all applicants must first have successfully completed a First Degree Reiki training course. Some schools and teachers will offer both First Degree and Second Degree Reiki training in one weekend module or other type of multi-day single session. However, most teachers will require a period of anywhere from 21 days to 3 months to have passed after completion of First Degree Reiki training to ensure the student has had time to adjust to the initial attunement and to have had plenty of practice with self-treatment.

The other reason for the required delay between First Degree and Second Degree training is that newly attuned students must be given the opportunity for their newly opened energy channels to establish themselves. Much of

Second Degree training involves additional attunements designed to open these channels even further, with a particular focus on the opening of the heart chakra. Typically, Second Degree training involves one additional attunement, though many teachers may provide several additional attunements during these sessions.

The attunements provided during Second Degree training increase the intensity of power and the amount of energy students will be able to access. The central channel will now be more fully opened, and Reiki will begin to flow more fully and steadily into the students' chakra systems.

Students at this level will also receive formal training in the use of hand positions, gassho meditation, Reiji-ho, and Chiryo, as well specific techniques such as Byosen scanning, in which the practitioner uses the Reiki flowing through his or hands to detect areas of stress in the patient's body and aura.

Finally, Second Degree Reiki training, students receive three "Reiki Symbols." The symbols each represent a different component of hos Reiki can be channeled and used to heal others. The three symbols received at this level are:

Power Symbol

The Japanese term for the Power Symbol is Cho Ku Ray, which has been translated as both, "I have the key," and "God and man coming together." The purpose of the power symbol is to allow the practitioner to increase the amount of Reiki to which he or she has access. By using the power symbol, the practitioner can open for close the connection to Reiki, thereby enabling the cleansing and purification of physical and energy spaces. To use the power symbol, the practitioner must draw the symbol over himself or herself and/or his or her patient and recite the words "Cho Ku Ray" three times, silently.

Mental Symbol

The Japanese term for the Mental Symbol is Sei Hei Ki, which has been translated as both, "The Key to the Universe," and, "God and man coming together." The mental symbol allows the practitioner to enter a different level of Reiki energy. Whereas the initial attunement allows the student to access mostly the physical healing aspects of Reiki, the mental symbol can allow him or her to transform this healing energy to address ailments associated with mental and emotional anguish and suffering. Once again, the practitioner must draw the symbol over himself or herself and his or her patient while reciting, "Sei Hei Ki." The Reiki energy will be attuned to address issues such as healing emotional or psychological trauma; emotional imbalances that result in unhealthy amounts of anger, sadness, or anxiety; helping patients remove blockages impairing their emotional function; and stopping habitual habits like smoking.

Distance Symbol

The Japanese term for this symbol is "Hon Sha Ze Sho Nen," which has been translated as, "The God in Me Greets the God In You to Promote Enlightenment and Peace." Students who have been attuned to this symbol in Second Degree training are able as practitioners to send healing over distances of time and space. When using the distance symbol, the patient does not need to be physically present; instead, the practitioner can draw the symbol and recite the phrase, "Hon Sha Ze Sho Nen," before transmitting the healing power of Reiki to an individual patient at a distant location. This symbol also works across time, allowing the practitioner to heal past traumas and wounds, or prepare participants in a future event to help ensure their success.

Third Degree Reiki/Reiki Master

The Japanese term for Third Degree Reiki training is Shinpiden. Third Degree training is sometimes combined with Master Level training.

During Third Degree training, students receive additional attunements to improve their ability to channel Reiki healing energy and to increase the power and intensity of that healing energy. In addition, Third Degree training requires students to focus more on spiritual healing components. Third Degree students will be better equipped to work with patients who complain about spiritual ailments. For this reason, the training at this level is also known as Inner Master training because it focuses students on developing an awareness that each of us is master of his or her own destiny. Third Degree students are better equipped to treat patients suffering from existential and spiritual crises by helping them find internal healing and direction. This use of Reiki healing is closer to the purposes and motivations of the founder, Dr. Mikao Usui.

Because of the difference in application and focus from Second to Third Degree, students are generally encouraged to wait a considerable amount of time between Second Degree and Third Degree training. After Second degree training, students should spend time gaining experience as practitioners and gain some degree of comfort and expertise in applying their skills as healers. The intense shift toward more spiritual and deeply personal healing benefits from time spent working at the Second Level.

Master Symbol

In addition, Third Degree students also receive the Master Symbol. The Japanese term for the Master Symbol is Dai Ki Myo, which has been translated as both, "Great Enlightenment," and, "Great Shining Light." The Master Symbol should be used by Third Degree students to establish a connection to the divine, and to facilitate healing at all levels.

Third Degree students who have been attuned to the Master Symbol are encouraged to invoke this symbol prior to all of their healing sessions. Invocation of this symbol, as with those others, requires drawing the symbol over oneself while reciting, "Dai Ki Myo." Invocation results in enhanced and more powerful healing across all forms of Reiki practice. Some examples of how Third Degree students use the Master Symbol include:

Enhancing the connection between the practitioner and Reiki to facilitate deep healing at the level of the soul.

Healing and opening of the chakras and the aura

Healing illness and disease from its original source at the level of the spiritual self.

Drawing out and releasing negative energy from both the physical body and spiritual energy body.

Developing and strengthening personal and spiritual growth and development, self-awareness, and intuition.

Increasing the ability of the healer to attain a higher state of enlightenment and become more psychic.

Strengthening of the immune system and increasing energy flow throughout the body.Enhancing the existing healing properties of herbs, medicines, or homeopathic remedies.Used in combination with other Reiki symbols, the Master Symbol can help increase the effectiveness of those symbols. For example, invoking the Master Symbol before using the Distance Symbol can speed the transfer of healing energy over distance.

Healers attuned to this symbol can purify and bring a higher dimension of light to all their healing practices.

Reiki Master

Finally, the Reiki Master level, which is sometimes combined with Third Degree training, is reserved for students who wish to become teachers to pass on the knowledge of Reiki to new practitioners. At the Master Level, students receive a Master attunement and training in how to attune others. This instruction in the attunement of others is what separates Master Level training form Third Degree training.

In addition, at the Master Level, there is generally an expectation of serious commitment from all students, and Master Level training explores more deeply and widely the varied applications of Reiki healing. For example, Tibetan Master Level training includes instruction in the use of four additional symbols—the Tibetan Master Symbols. Reiki Masters are uniquely equipped not only to provide a wide array of highly specialized healing practices to treat many types of illnesses and diseases, but also to train new students and to conduct their own journeys of self-discovery with renewed insight.

Chapter 5.
Healing Ailments

On the surface or skin of every living being, there's some energy that surrounds them. More like a magnetic field but swap magnet for energy. This energy is called an aura. It does not just float around the surface of the body; some of it seeps into the body too.

The intensity of an aura is different for each person depending on a lot of reasons like mood, the environment, and so on.

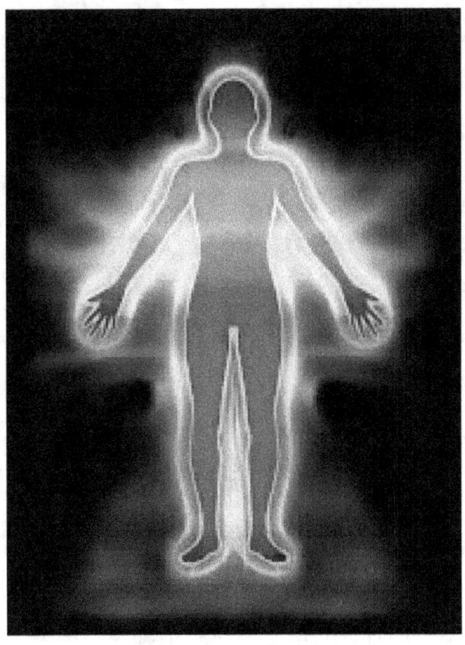

All the layers constantly affect the emotional, mental, physical, and spiritual state of a person, as well as the people around them. What I'm saying is that if one teeny tiny layer of your aura is wonky, your whole aura may get wonky too. The layers are connected to every chakra in the body. Please don't make me explain chakras again.

Aura levels and your corresponding needs

1) **Vital level** - Rational mind. To understand the situation in a clear, linear, rational way.

2) **The ethereal level** - Emotions with respect to self. Self-acceptance and self-love.

3) **Spiritual level** - Divine mind, serenity. To be connected to divine mind and to understand the greater universal pattern.

4) **Astral level** - Relations with others. Loving interaction with friends and family.

5) **Lower mental level** - Divine will within. To align with the divine will within, to make a commitment to speak and follow the truth.

6) **Higher mental level** - Divine love, and spiritual ecstasy.

Aura colors and their meaning

<u>Blue aura</u> Unfortunately, blue isn't just blue. There is dark blue, light blue, turquoise blue, yada yada yada. And each shade of blue means something in the aura world. Dark blue means psychic or clairvoyant. Turquoise blue means bad energy. If your aura is turquoise blue, it means you are empathic, and likely have attracted the negative energies of the people around you.

Red Aura Bright red is typically like the turquoise aura in relation to empathy. Light red aura means you're positive and full of energy! But people with this aura are good at using smiles to cover up a bucket load of tears. Dark red means bad energy or negative feelings. You need to let the past go.

Green aura Light green stands for healing and compassion. But people with this aura usually don't take part in things that don't particularly concern them. They'd rather not waste their time. This can be a good thing and a bad thing. Dark green represents negativity like other dark colours I mentioned. Anger and jealousy is usually associated with this aura. Green-eyed monster!

Pink aura When people think pink, they think soft, feminine, right? If you have a pink aura, you're not so different from people with a red aura. You're just purer. Like other aura, the pink aura has different shades. Baby pink aura means you're not materialistic. You don't care about Fendi, Lambos or Kylie Jenner. Bright pink aura represents a balance between the spiritual world and the material world. It is an updated baby pink version. Dark pink aura means you're slowly finding yourself on the path of negativity but you're still pink, so it's not too late to fix it.

White aura You guessed it! It represents purity. Not much talk there.

Purple aura If you have this aura, you probably just love love and relationships. This color is linked to the heart chakra which explains a lot.

Black aura First of all, this aura doesn't automatically scream evil. It might mean chaos and turmoil or just a blocked aura.

Yellow aura This aura has connections to life energy and the spleen. It is the color of intelligence, spiritual awakening, inspiration, creativity, joy and sheer happiness. Just like other auras, this one also has different shades that represent different things. Light or pale yellow represents spiritual and psychic awareness. Hope. Positivity. New ideas.

If you seem to be struggling to maintain control over a relationship or you have a major fear of not being in control, your aura is most definitely bright lemon-yellow. If it's a shiny metallic gold, you are full of inspiration, spirituality, and power. Dark yellow or brown? Students most likely have this aura because of the fatigue and excessive studying trying to cover the entire curriculum.

Gold aura This is the color of enlightenment and protection from a higher power. Whenever you see this aura is a person, know that he/she is protected by a divine power. It signifies wisdom, deep knowledge, spirituality, intuition, and divinity.

Crystals are beautiful naturally occurring stones with a lot of amazing properties and uses. Crystals are a big part of unorthodox medicine, a good example being Reiki.

These chakras are like passageways, and when there's a roadblock, energy won't be able to spread to necessary parts of the body. A million things can cause a chakra roadblock.

Some crystals happen to exist to unblock chakras, among

other things. These crystals can be placed in the area of the chakra blockage during a Reiki session or held in the hand of the patient.

It's important to note that not all crystals unblock all chakras. Each chakra has its own specific set of crystals, so a third eye chakra gemstone cannot unblock your throat chakra. Mostly these gemstones are associated with the chakras by color except for a select few. We may have covered a few already, but I'm going to go over a few more attributes, okay?

Let's take a look shall we?

• Aquamarine Crystal

Aquamarine is a big deal in the energy stone business and a great healing companion to Reiki. It is the stone for you if you are seeking courage, determination, strength, success and communication.

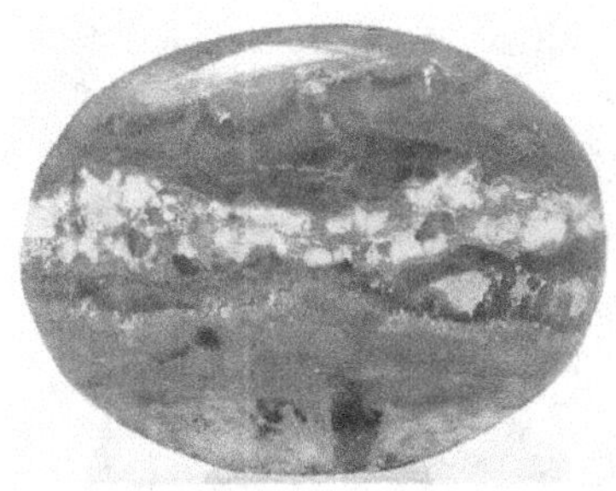

Because it is an ocean stone, it provides calm to whoever possesses it. It is really useful during meditation or yoga for clarity, creativity and self-expression. Aquamarine is also believed to protect those who travel on water. Buy a bracelet or necklace with aquamarine crystals.

This stone will help reduce anxiety and depression. It is a throat chakra crystal and it enhances speech and honesty. Aquamarine is an excellent stone for reaching the highest level of your spirituality while keeping yourself well-grounded at the same time.

• Rhodonite Crystal

Rhodonite is a beautiful red stone that is linked to the heart chakra. This is used to treat emotional wounds and past scars and even physical wounds. However, when you have serious physical injuries, this stone won't stitch you up nicely, so tell a friend to get you an Uber cause honey, you need a doctor.

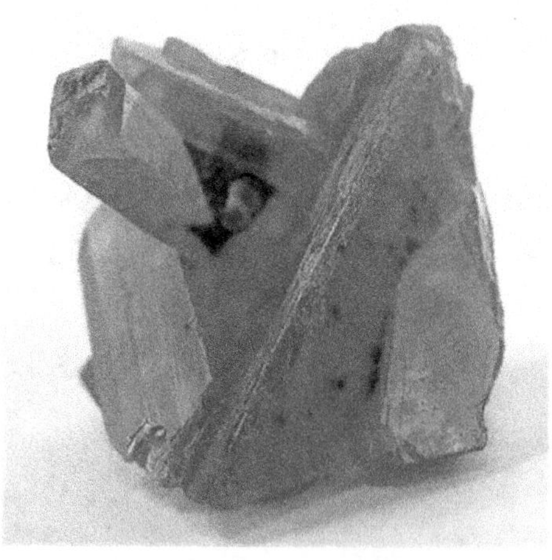

After you get medical care however, you can place the rhodonite gem on the area to speed up healing.

Rhodonite is the stone of love, empathy and affection, being connected with the heart chakra and all. It maintains the balance between good and evil. When there's an issue of panic attack, abuse and dependency, use this stone.

• Selenite Crystal

Selenite is a Crown chakra stone and is great for Reiki healing because of the many ways it can be helpful to physical and spiritual health. It is sometimes called the calming stone because it is used to calm people during Reiki sessions or meditation.

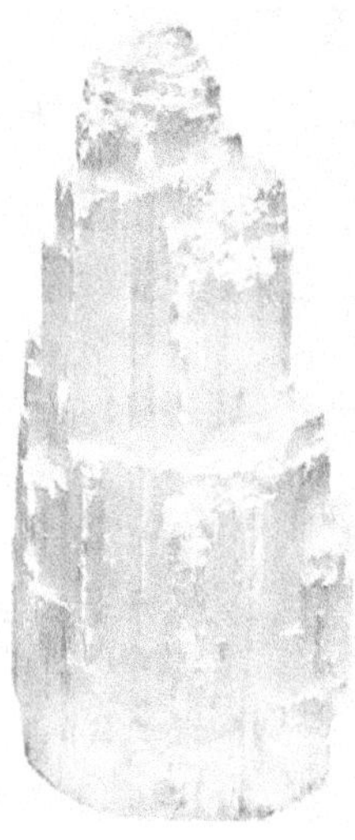

In meditation, it reveals your inner truth and relaxes your troubled mind. It is used for mental enhancement, telepathy and astral projection. Selenite is a self-cleansing stone. Put selenite in your room to disperse negative energy.

• Clear quartz

Clear quartz is a crown chakra crystal that deals with storage, absorption and regulation of energy.

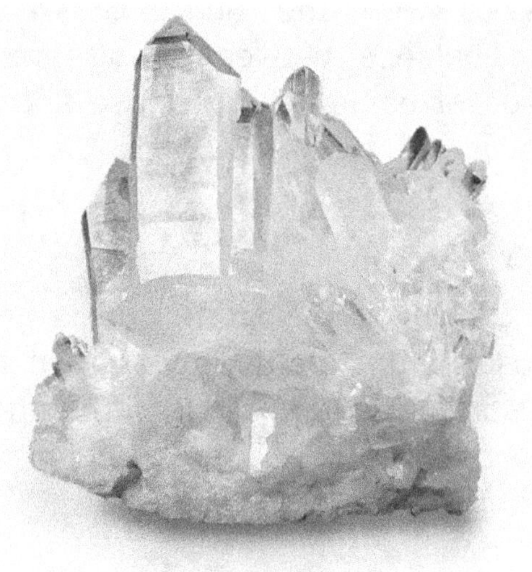

This stone attracts negative energy and draws it out of our bodies and environments. It is a purification stone.

• Amethyst Crystal

Amethyst is known to be very protective. It increases your energy to a level where negative energies cannot reach and hurt you. This stone is a protection stone with calming properties.

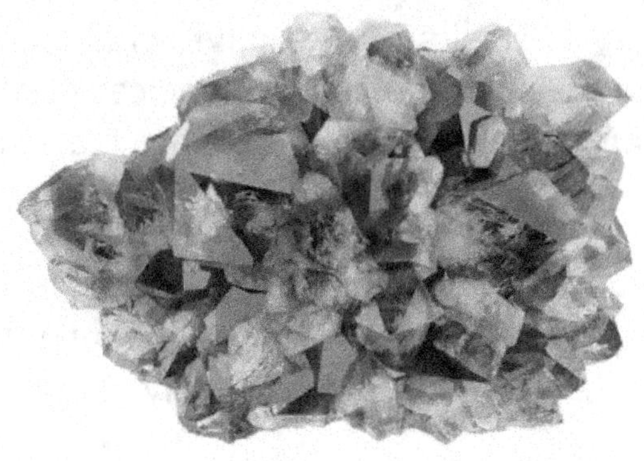

Use this stone during Reiki to create a beautiful combination of love and healing energies. Amethyst helps with sleeping problems, stress, migraines and paranoia.

• Red Jasper Crystal

Red jasper, a gem usually associated with the root chakra energy, is one of the most effective stones for the protection of your own energy system when you are surrounded by negative energies of any kind.

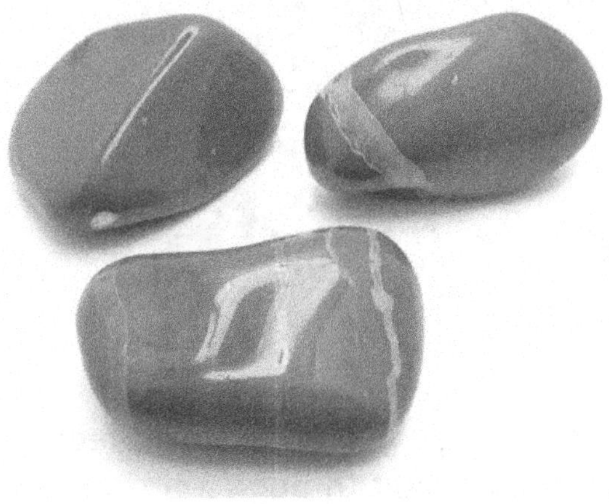

What's more, red jasper gives you the courage to speak up. It is a very helpful stone to have with you if you find yourself between a rock and a hard place. Red jasper can also heal your aura and balance out your energies by filtering the negative ones.

Whenever you are surrounded by a negative energy, red jasper will draw it out of the environment into itself. It will literally take the hit and most likely crack or split into pieces.

• Tiger eye Crystal

This beautiful stone is also known as the shape-shifting stone. It builds courage and stability. When you use this stone during a Reiki session, you will find your confidence has been given an immense boost.

This is the gemstone of the solar plexus chakra, and we all know what this chakra is about, don't we?

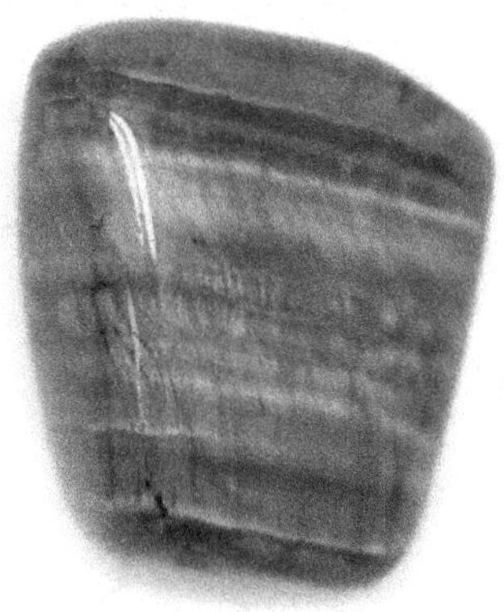

The tiger stone helps get rid of toxic feelings, fear, and self-doubt. Try holding it through a horror movie... ha!

If you find yourself drowning in self-doubt, hold this stone in your hand and imagine its energy flowing through your solar plexus chakra.

• Bloodstone Crystal

Bloodstone energy is the kind that hits you like a proper workout or a fun date. it's plain amazing! Bloodstone touches every single cell of your body so that you're not just living, you are bursting with life!

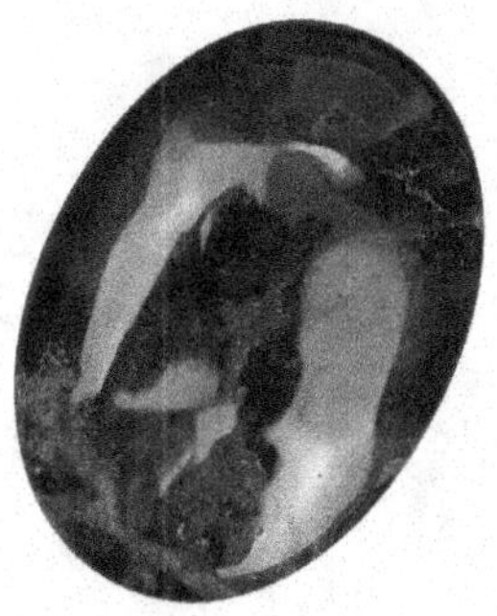

When you need a reminder of what gets your blood racing - in a good way - in life, get in sync with the energy this stone. Bloodstone healing is all about getting you up and about. This is not a stone that allows you stay right where you are.

With this stone, time in your comfort zone is limited. You have to be on the go! If you're feeling lazy or just uninterested, bloodstone will snap you right out of it. This is particularly useful if you're taking on a new project.

This stone is a heart chakra stone as you may have already guessed, and it is used to open up the heart to feel and love again. This stone will give you the strength and courage to go back out there and start doing the things you love!

• **Flower Agate Crystal**

Flower Agate is a brand-new stone all the way from Madagascar. Like a blossom tree, this gemstone will help you bloom into your greatest potential. This is a stone of transformation, new beginnings and growth.

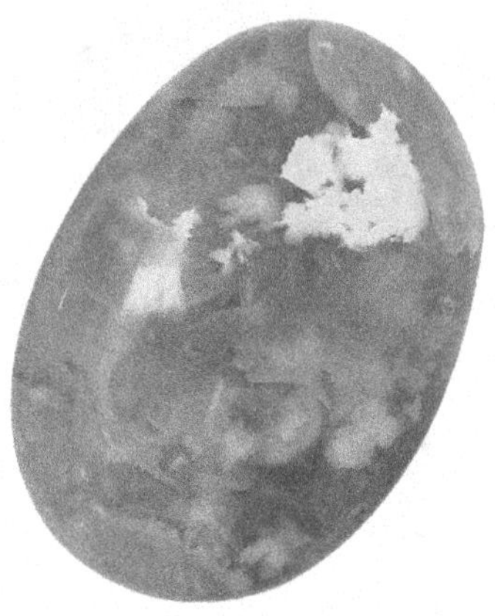

This cherry-like stone will fill you with joy and revival. Imagine running around through a field of sunflowers with no shoes on. Pure freedom, am I right? Wear jewelry with this stone when you are seeking love and transformation. During Reiki, you could place it anywhere on your body or just hold it in your palm. If life's got you down, get a flower agate ASAP!

Every day, we are exposed to other people and their various energies, and sometimes, they may not be carrying the best of energies. When we become exposed to their toxic energies, we may end up ill or worse. Because usually, even a disease as tiny as a cold can be caused by a blocked chakra or absorbing a negative energy.

More often than not, we need to take a break from all this energy overload and take care to cleanse our auras. Inviting random and not so random people into your home leaves you susceptible to a lot of things, because they might leave pieces of their energies behind and those tiny bits of energy need to be purged.

Other reasons to cleanse your space include but are not limited to the following:

- Psychic blood suckers. There are some people who love dragging people down their large black hole of despair. They usually don't like empaths and look the other way when they come across one. These people can drain the life and joy out of you just like vampires, but this time, it's not your blood, it's your energy.
- Visitors. Your home is pretty much your temple. It is a very sacred place and should be treated as such. Personally, I don't like having a lot of people over because my home is my safe haven. It's a place I go to recharge.

When people come into my home, they leave specs of their energies on my couch, floor, door handle, everywhere! And I have to cleanse for my safety and the safety of those closest to me. Your home should be your comfort zone, your sensitive place too and when you have people over, you should cleanse the environment because you want the vibe of your home to match your personal energy. Think of cleansing like adjusting the temperature of your air conditioner. I'm not saying neve have visitors. I'm saying you should take care of your safe space.

You're probably wondering how to cleanse and protect yourself because you can't avoid people until you die. Well, you can build a shield or force field around yourself with certain protective crystals in the form of house decor or jewellery.

Setting boundaries can save you a lot of trouble and stress. Think of it like drawing a line with chalk around yourself or going into a personal invincible bubble to keep from drama and stress. Boundaries are not complicated at all, not like literal walls anyway.

How to Protect Yourself with Reiki

Depending on your level in the Reiki business, you can use Reiki symbols. You could draw your symbols around you as if you are in an invisible bubble. You could say the names of the symbols at random times during your day. Draw the same symbols on top of your head, and underneath your feet.

Some people prefer the Reiki Box shaped protection. I usually recommend the egg shape, since it matches the shape of the aura. However, you can use both for different purposes whenever you like. If you are not really attuned to Reiki, or if you are still at Reiki level one, you can protect yourself by imagining white or golden light around you while meditating. I also recommend working with angels, and different Reiki colors. The color for Reiki protection is a deep violet. You can try various colors for specific protection, or to invite different angels into your home or personal space.

Cleansing Your Home

Step 1: Light your candle or candles and some sage on your altar or anywhere really. Feel free to substitute sage for incense or something else, as long as you know it's intended to cleanse. Relax, take some deep breaths before you begin. I usually state my intentions for my cleansing, and 'activate' the Reiki energy within me. Depending on what system of Reiki you use, use the form you find most comfortable. If you are not attuned to Reiki, that's okay, just pray, state your intentions for your space cleansing, and ask your angels for assistance.

Step 2: Start by spreading the sage around yourself. Go on, breathe it in, and move it all around your body, both front and back. Now you can start with the room you are currently in and try drawing the Reiki symbols on each wall of that room. You can use any symbols you like. As you do this, be sure to speak your cleansing intentions out loud for what you want in your space. Usually, I find myself banishing negative energies from my space, and inviting angels to stay with me here in my home. I don't know about you. Do this for all the rooms if you feel it is necessary. Depending on the frequency of your cleansings, you may only want to cleanse specific rooms. Remember to always cleanse your doorways, particularly the entrances to your home. The negative energy most likely goes through there.

Step 3: Now that you're done cleansing and sanctifying, place your sage down. Be thankful to your angels. Ask your angels & guides to keep watching and protecting you, guiding you, and fighting for you. Pray as much as you need, no time limit there. Take a deep breath in your new space, and trust me, it will feel brand new, as if you opened up a window and fresh air and positivity came through. Bask in it, love!

Whether you are into Reiki healing or empathic healing, you may be picking up energies from other people throughout the day unknowingly. Knowing how to cleanse yourself and your home is a very important survival skill.

Chapter 6.
The Five Reiki Principles

When Dr Usui taught Reiki, he took a holistic view and taught not only Reiki healing but also Reiki as an opportunity for spiritual development and personal growth. Coming from a Buddhist background and perspective, Dr Usui believed that constant progress towards enlightenment was just as important as - or perhaps even more important than - purely physical healing.

As well as the essential Reiki hand positions, symbols and techniques, he would teach his students a range of spiritual practices and philosophies, with the aim of helping them to develop themselves as well-rounded individuals, and to subsequently become better healers.

Among the philosophies, spiritual practices and ideologies shared and taught along with the Reiki healing system, were the following five Reiki principles:

Just for today, I will not worry

Just for today, I will not be angry

Just for today, I will be grateful

Just for today, I will work hard on myself

Just for today, I will be kind to every living thing

Dr Usui told his students that these were principles for Reiki practitioners to live by, in order to live happy and fulfilled lives. Over the years, there has been a great deal of debate about their correct translation and meaning, and you will find a bewildering number of slight modifications and variations online. Meditate on them and see which ones feel useful and resonant for you, and feel free to choose your own version from the ones available. There is no dogma in Reiki, just trust what you feel.

Here are some of the things I understand from the version I have chosen to share with you here. Please do your own research and check in with your heart in order to understand their meaning personally, and on a deeper level.

Each of the principles begins with the words, "Just for today..." I remember years ago posting the Reiki principles on Facebook, in order to share them with others. The responses that came back were incredibly judgmental about the words "Just for today". People wanted to know why just for today, why not every day. They filled up that comment feed with a whole load of shoulds, shoulding all over what I consider to be the real beauty and wisdom of these principles.

I find the "Just for today.." affirmation to be one of the wisest and most profound aspects of the Reiki principles, because it allows for human frailty, and is therefore based in reality and compassionate understanding of the human condition, rather than piety and pretence. In these days of instant gratification and misrepresentation, it's all too easy for any one of us to post a pretty picture quote on social media about being good, patient and kind, when that's what we're feeling in that brief moment. But if, five minutes later, we're getting annoyed with someone for not doing their washing up or for playing their music too loudly, or jumping the queue in the supermarket, the wisdom of our post will have expired within minutes.

Dr Usui recognised and acknowledged that the journey towards enlightenment and a peaceful spirit was a human journey, and that, as human beings, we were bound to fail or be utterly miserably if we constantly set ourselves unrealistic goals for self-development. He knew that the journey to Nirvana was a one day at a time thing! So, he gave us freedom to take it one day at a time. Just for today, I will not anger... is, for most of us at least, an achievable goal. When we reach it, we feel a great sense of achievement; while striving towards it we are able to remain mindful of it, minute by minute; and when we fail, we can try again tomorrow... and the next day.

Just for today, I will not worry

How many times has worrying robbed you of your peace in the moment, only to be exposed as fruitless when things turn out to be okay after all?! Worrying solves nothing and always robs us of our peace. If we are natural and compulsive worriers, worrying can take days, or even weeks away from us and in the end, when we look back, we often discover that it was all for nothing. When we let go of worry, we are more connected to higher consciousness because we are demonstrating trust in the divine plan, and this in turn inspires us with more confidence. When we worry, we are essentially saying that we don't trust the divine Power that runs through everything. This world-shaping Power is the exact same force that runs through us when we activate our Reiki channels. Worrying things will always happen, but if we are working with Reiki energy daily and making it an integral part of our spiritual work, why would we ever need to worry?!

Just for today, I will not be angry

Although anger is a very natural response in many situations, as Reiki practitioners and spiritual seekers, it's important for us to be able to notice our anger and set daily intentions to refrain from reacting angrily. Just as worrying things will always happen, so too will things that make us angry. There are times when the world seems to be a very fraught and angry place, however, it's important for us to remember that we also have access to the energy that created the universe. The Divine Reiki energy that flows through us can be called upon throughout the day, when we feel in need of comfort, understanding and emotional balance. Getting angry disrupts our emotional balance and, as healers, we can maintain a stronger connection to that divine presence when we refuse to react to incendiary situations and learn to reflect, re-connect and respond instead. And even if we find it impossible to remain calm every single day of our lives, with the energy of Reiki to sooth us and calm our nerves and tempers, most of us can honestly say, just for today, I will not get angry.

Just for today, I will be grateful

Gratitude is essential for opening our hearts. When we feel unhappy, it is often because we are focusing on all the negative things in our lives, and feeling unable to appreciate the good. When this lack of gratitude continues over time, we may become depressed and depleted. A lack of gratitude lowers our vibration, and in order to become consistently happy and remain clear channels for Reiki, it's important for us to find, on a daily basis, several reasons to be grateful. "Just for today, I will be grateful" could be adhered to simply by keeping a gratitude journal and writing down five things each day for which we are truly grateful.

Just for today, I will work hard on myself

There is often a variation on this particular principle, which I have also seen translated and interpreted as: Just for today, I will earn an honest living. However, there are many Reiki masters who believe that the translation is much closer to, Just for today, I will work hard, and that the 'work' to which Dr. Usui was referring was the work we do on ourselves to achieve spiritual progression and eventually enlightenment.

Both translations are important. Obviously, as spiritual beings and practitioners of a spiritual modality, we want to also live with a high degree of integrity and live in an honest way that feels good to us within our hearts. This also keeps our energy vibration high and clear. But, once again, it's important to remember that Dr Usui was a devoutly spiritual man and would always encourage his students to not only work on others but to also commit daily time and effort to the pursuit of spiritual development.

I have seen from personal experience that daily spiritual practice can yield innumerable rewards and benefits, but it's not always possible to maintain a rigorous daily scheduled of personal development, meditation, yoga, chanting, self-examination and any number of the wide variety of tools available to us. However, right now, in this moment - Just for today - we can all commit to doing one thing that enhances our spiritual progression or keeps us mindful of our evolutionary path. Dr Usui believed that working hard on ourselves should always be a priority, and that if we all worked hard on ourselves and allowed Reiki to transform us, the world would eventually also be transformed and become a much better place.

Just for today, I will be kind to every living thing

As healers and spiritual seekers, it's important for us to expand our desire to do good, by attempting to bring healing into all of our encounters with others in the wider world. There's no point connecting with this beautiful energy for the purpose of improving the life conditions of a handful of people, when we treat the rest of the world unkindly. Reiki is not only a practice, it is also a consciousness, and a pledge to move through the world seeking to do only good, and to share the healing vibration of this beautiful energy and practice. And, of course, the best teacher is the example we set in the world.

Being kind to every living thing doesn't mean allowing ourselves to be taken advantage of. Being kind can mean seeing things from a higher perspective and trying to understand why certain people behave the way they do, rather than becoming angry or defensive. The more we connect with the Reiki energy, the more we become able to see the higher perspective. We may even receive psychic insights about others which allow us to become even more compassionate towards them. We might see glimpses of their past lives or even lives we have shared with them, and often when we gain these higher perspectives, we begin to see others much more through the eyes of love, or through Reiki-eyes, always attempting to develop a Reiki spirit that permeates everything we do.

In other words, giving someone a Reiki treatment and then kicking the cat is not consistent energy. It's like becoming a vegan to save the animals and the planet, and then making endless angry videos about meat-eaters .and other vegans who are not strict enough. At some point the loving-kindness needs to penetrate into our souls. Being kind means trying to find the balance and compassion in our hearts that allows us to love others unconditionally, and to be channels of Reiki all day, every day, flooding the world with this wonderful heart-centred awareness. This way, we always leave people and situations in a much better state than when we first found them, and increase our own capacity to remain in a happier state.

Being kind to every living thing and seeing the higher perspective doesn't mean, however, that we should remain in abusive situations or tolerate abuse in any form. Sometimes we learn a very hard lesson this way. Being a healer doesn't mean we can fix everyone, in fact, it's not our job to fix everyone... Always be humble enough to remember that there is a higher plan for every one of us. Being kind also means being kind to ourselves, and being wise enough to step aside and allow divine love to do the work when we are not able to.

There may be times when we don't feel like being kind, for example, when circumstances force us to live with unpleasant or unreasonable people, but it's important to remember, even in the midst of these difficult times that everything teaches us something and, in each moment, even if we know with all our hearts that we are in the presence of people we cannot possibly tolerate for a lifetime, we can certainly awaken each day with the resolute intention that, Just for today, we will be as kind as humanly possible, and endeavour to bring peace and happiness to ourselves, to others and to the wider world, no matter what. Even when you're packing your bags in secret and arranging therapy to heal your addiction to abusive partners, you can smile inwardly as you dream of your new life, and say quietly within your heart, "Just for today, I will be kind to every living thing."

Chapter 7.
Reiki and Crystals

Are you familiar with crystal healing? At the very least, you must be familiar with the glittering stones used in jewelry and decorative purposes. Other than this, crystals are also used for various technical and scientific purposes.

There are hundreds of different crystals available for you to use. Every crystal is unique in how it looks and its intrinsic properties. Each crystal can be used for different purposes as they have different properties that will work for different concerns. If you combine crystal healing with Reiki, the strength of the healing will be further enhanced. Two natural energy sources will be combined in this process, and it will help you heal more effectively and at a much faster rate.

If your Reiki practitioner decides to use crystals during the Reiki session, they will use the ones that are most appropriate for whatever ailment or concern you have. One of the most commonly used methods is the crystal layout. A normal Reiki-receiving session will involve you lying down on a flat surface. With crystals involved, the healer will place the right crystals on your body. Every point in your body is associated with different concerns, and the crystals will be placed accordingly. After the crystals are placed, the healer will continue with the Reiki session as per usual; however, now you will get the added strength of the crystal energy too. When the Reiki energy and crystal energy combine, any blockage within you can be cleared. It will help the energy flow freely through you and maintain a healthy balance within your chakras as well. Reiki with crystals will help you deal with any energy, spiritual, or emotional block that ails you.

Being aware of what your body tells you is important. Reiki will help you in increasing this self-awareness. You will be able to identify any point in your body that feels weak or hurt. You or the healer can then use the correct crystals that help to treat those regions. This will help to identify the correct chakra that is out of balance as well. Crystals can be placed on the energy center concerned and with Reiki; the chakras can be realigned properly again.

Using crystals while receiving Reiki will help you in feeling more energized and rejuvenated. Certain crystals will fill you with confidence and motivation. Use your self-awareness to identify the emotions that need to be dealt with. Then use the related crystals that help to transform negative emotions into positive ones. You will be able to find the cause of a problem and bring balance back into your body. Using crystals with Reiki can enhance your overall state of well-being and aid significantly in the healing process.

Reiki Session with Crystals

Have you ever tried a Reiki session combined with the use of crystals? Well, here you will learn what you can expect if you do. Usually, the healer will ask you to lie down on your back on a comfortable flat surface like most other Reiki sessions. The Reiki will help you reach a state of deep relaxation. A grounding crystal is usually placed near the feet, and then the healer will place other crystals in the appropriate regions of your body.

The placement of the crystals is usually done from the feet to the head. The healer needs to have sufficient knowledge about crystal healing so that they know which crystals should be used and where they need to be placed. It is important for you to inform them clearly about what your main issues are so they know what needs to be dealt with. When the crystals have been placed on the body, the healer will continue with the Reiki session.

Energy will pass into you from the crystals as well as the hands of the healer as they give you Reiki. This energy will pass onto the energy centers of all the chakras and help to keep them balanced. You will notice that the session leaves you feeling completely relaxed and at peace. Towards the end of the session, the healer will start removing all the crystals, starting from your head to the ones at your feet. You will notice that the placement of crystals at the beginning is from the bottom to the top while removal is the opposite way.

Another thing to notice is that the healer will not rush any part of the process; everything will be carried out calmly and with patience. After the session, the healer will also guide you and tell you how you can practice Reiki with crystals by yourself to further heal you.

Examples of Some Crystals You Can Use

Selenite

It works as a cleansing crystal and can be used to recharge other crystals as well. Selenite can work like a conduit that will help you achieve a deeper level of consciousness as you reach out to the universe and your inner self. It also has a connecting power between the spiritual world and this dimension. This crystal will help to heal and bring inner peace when used during meditation.

Moonstone

It is a crystal that will strengthen your intuition and help to bring harmony. Carry this crystal to help you in removing materialistic behavior and living a better life that will support the purpose of Reiki. This stone also helps to treat indigestion and hormonal imbalances.

Citrine

This crystal is believed to be related to wealth in most parts of the world. If you want to attract financial wealth, then use this stone. It will also help to restore stability if you have any monetary issues. Other than money, this crystal promotes better digestion, improved mental capacity, and better nervous system functioning.

Rose Quartz

One of the most commonly used crystals, rose quartz is linked to love. If you want to attract love or need help to improve your relationships with others, use this crystal. It also helps you personally in healing from any emotional wounds and helps you transition from a negative state of mind to a positive one.

Opal

It is a beautiful stone which displays different colors under rays of light. Opal is linked to your third-eye chakra and amplifies vibrant energy in you. It is used for inspiring optimism and happiness in a person. Healthwise, this stone is considered helpful to treat any ailments of the eye. It also has a stimulatory effect on your memory.

There are so many other crystals that you can use and learn more about. Each will help you in a distinctly different way. You should also accept that a crystal has to be right for you in order for it to work. Don't just pick a random crystal; take time and see which connects to you. Choosing a crystal that has a real connection with you will make it much more effective. Crystal healing is another alternative healing tool that you should explore along with Reiki to get better results. You can use a crystal in so many ways. Just carry it with you in your pocket or wear it as a ring or pendant. You can keep crystals in your home or at work as well to spread positive energy. The most effective and proactive way to harness the energy of crystals will be during the practice of Reiki. So go ahead and explore something new; you won't regret it.

Chapter 8.
Reiki And Body Energy

Everything is about energy, which means that healing also ultimately involves energy. In Reiki, energy helps promote healing through enhancing the flow of energy and correcting any disturbances that occur in the "human energy field," also called the aura. This aura permeates the body and surrounds it. When the body experiences the flow of energy, the body will have the capacity to heal by itself.

Energy healing works on the basis that your body is made up of various patterns of energy. When you work directly with body energy, you will influence the mental, physical, and emotional level. Using energy healing in Reiki is seen to be holistic in nature.

This is why it is vital that when your body or mind experiences disturbances, everyone wants to address these levels. However, energy healing doesn't work on its own; rather, it supports other healing methods that we use in daily life. Reiki healing focuses on the energy of which your body, mind, and emotions are made up of.

At the center of the human field are seven primary chakras that are supported by thousands of other smaller meridians and chakras. The seven chakras are placed in a vertical manner along your spinal column, and it begins on the pelvic floor. The first one is the Root chakra that is at the level of the pelvic bone, and the one at the top is the Crown chakra. Each of the chakras works as its own transmitter as well as the recipient of the energy. When the chakra receives the energy, it will direct it to corresponding organs as well as the endocrine system within the body.

The Energetic Bodies

In addition to the chakra, the human body uses the human energy field to make it work perfectly. The energy field is made up of smaller energetic bodies, which include the mental, spiritual, etheric, emotional, and physical bodies. All these allow you to relate with and experience the environment in different aspects.

When all the chakras and energy bodies are in harmony and are working well together, you will be full of vitality and have a sense of wellness. On the other hand, when the energy centers are not balanced, you will become sluggish, and you will experience confusion, fatigue, and illness at all times. You need to work with a healing practice that can identify the problem areas. He will do so with the aim of releasing the blockages then create a positive flow of energy in the body so that he can make you heal. Healing can happen immediately, or it can take time.

The 5 Layers of the Human Energy Field

As described earlier, the human energy field is composed of 5 layers that we explore below:

Physical Energy

This is the layer that we look at to be the physical part of ourselves. Although we look at the body as a package that consists of the skin, flesh, bones, and organs, they also have energy, similar to the other layers of the body that you can't see, or you cannot sense such as the mind.

Etheric

This word is derived from the word "ether," – which is a layer that sits from one quarter to one half of an inch, but not any more than an inch, from the location of the physical body. The practitioners that have sensed this body describe it as a feeling that is gray in color. It is like a spider web, and it can stretch, and it is usually seen as the blueprint of the physical layer.

Emotional Energy

This is the third layer from the outside. It is at the center of all the five layers that we have looked at. The emotional layer is the layer where fears and feelings reside. It can be very volatile when we have emotions. It comes into play whether you are experiencing both low and high emotions.

Mental Energy

This is the layer where our ideas and other emotions spring from. It also forms the store from which the belief system gets stored. This is the space where our thoughts are stored then sorted out, and it is where people store their personal truths or any perceptions that are based on experiences.

Spiritual Energy

This is the final layer, where higher awareness and consciousness is stored. It is the layer where our past lives are tied as well as the universal consciousness that is common to all people.

Why Should You Be Concerned About Energy Field?

Studies show that the main factor that will limit you is the low-frequency energies that you have stored within your body. You need to be aware that the personal energy field has a huge impact on the general sense of well-being. People are usually aware of how important personal hygiene is. You need to know that the physical body gets dirty when you use it, and it can pick up viruses and bacteria that can lead to disease. So, if you stop looking after your body, your physical health, as well as a sense of well-being, will also suffer.

Have you ever felt that your state of mind feels "dirty" when your body is dirty as well? This is because everything that you do is connected to the energy, which also means that every part of your life comes with an energy component. Visible dirt is just a part of the bigger problem. Any part of your body is made up of many energy frequencies, most that cannot be seen with the naked eye. However, you need to know that the unseen energy frequencies will affect the energy field as well.

The major problem that we face is that we have grown up in a society that doesn't acknowledge the unseen energies and how they are important to our lives. In school, we are only taught about the energies that we can see, and how they affect our lives, we aren't taught about what we cannot see.

For you to understand how it all works, you need to look at all the five layers of the human energy fields. It is a fact that for you to have total body hygiene, you ought to keep all the five layers of body energy clean. When you have knowledge about the different fields, you will be able to know that the conditions in your body that you think is caused by physical causes might be due to energy imbalance. You don't need to limit yourself at a single part of the body; rather, you need to look at the different layers before you make any conclusion. So, if you wish to handle the proper healing of the body, you need to do so by working at all the layers of the body.

Energy Healing: What You Need to Know

When you go through the paces of energy healing, you need to make sure that you understand what has been done before and what else needs to be done. Here are the top things that you need to understand about energy healing:

1. It has Been Studied for Many Years

Reiki has been used in traditional Japanese medicine for many years. Additionally, Chakras have been described in ancient Hindu scripts. Acupuncture uses the meridians to find healing power. We can see that ancient cultures used these different modalities to stimulate your body's natural ability to heal and be better. They identified internal energy as the best way to heal the whole body.

2. It Is Based on Science

In physics class in high school, we learned that matter is composed of molecules that are in constant motion. Even something that is as solid as a rock is also vibrating continuously. People that have a fulfilling life vibrate at a higher frequency compared to people with low frequency. Places also have vibration frequencies as well. When the place has a vibe, it will either give you a positive or a negative vibe as well. Places that have a negative vibe will make it impossible for you to be in the space for long. For instance, air at the beach is at a higher frequency, which makes it easy for you to sit and relax.

3. Energy Healing Is for Everyone

You don't need to grasp the concept of energy healing in order for you to enjoy the benefits. When you decide to try it out, make sure you go with an open mind so that you enjoy all the benefits. You can visit an energy healer any time you like. If you are anxious or stressed, a session with an energy healer is ideal for you. The session will help you feel more balanced and relax, as well. If you are already feeling so good, you will get to feel better when you use the method of energy healing. However, we need to stress that energy healing is an alternative form of healing. You need to combine it with other conventional medical procedures to achieve total healing.

4. It Is Accessible

You can work with Reiki healers the world over. Many people think that Reiki healers are just confined to a certain part of the world, but this is a wrong notion. The truth is that you can get a healer right to your doorstep; all you need to do is to find a way to link up with them. Do you know that you can make use of Reiki healing even without meeting the healer face to face? Yes, it is true. All you need to know is that the power of Reiki can make the energy to flow to where it is required. For the most part, you need to get referrals from people that have used the practice before for it to be successful. Ask a friend who is into energy healing or ask your yoga master at the studio for referrals.

5. You Can Connect with Your Inner Self at Home

Just the way you wake up each morning and brush your teeth, you can also make healing your daily habit so that you enjoy the various benefits. Once you have a session with the energy healer, you can keep the energy flowing by using homemade energy healing remedies such as taking a bath with Epsom salts each day. All you need to experience the healing powers of your energy is to be willing to learn and to start on the journey to wellness.

Chapter 9.
Attunements

Reiki attunements are a powerful spiritual initiation. This is the heart of Reiki. The attunement energy is divinely inspired and originates from Divine Source itself. The Reiki attunement is a transfer of energy through the Master to the student with the attunement being given by the Reiki Master's guides in spirit. It aligns the student with the Universal Life Force Energy of Reiki and allows Reiki energy to channel through the body of the student.

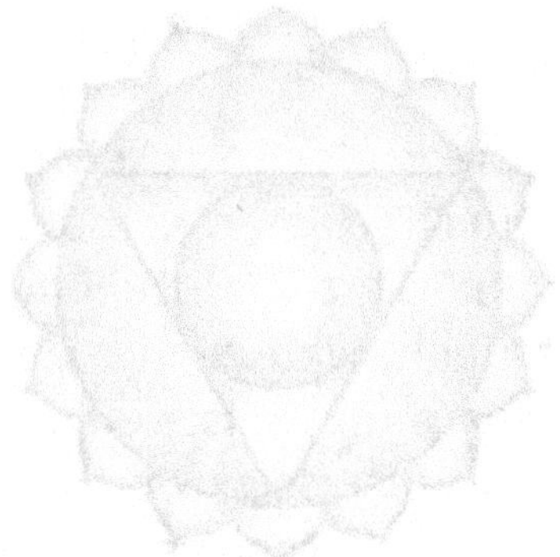

What To Expect

Normally students are seated in a chair for the attunement. The student begins with their hands in prayer position over their Heart Chakra. I like to smudge my student with sage smoke (if they have agreed first that this is something they would like). The student is instructed to keep their eyes closed during the entire attunement process. If they are very uncomfortable with this, they can focus straight ahead at a crystal or candle flame. The student is instructed to imagine Reiki energy flowing through them, coming down from their Crown Chakra, running through their body, and expanding out into their aura.

Group or Individual

I personally prefer to perform individual attunements. I take each student into a separate area where I give them their attunement. Some Masters attune their students in groups where the students are lined up in rows or in a small circle. If attunements are given in a group and some are attuned before the others are finished, all must remain in quiet meditation until the whole group is finished.

Distant Attunements

Although most people prefer to receive their attunement in person with a Reiki Master, a student can also be attuned through a distant attunement. I do this occasionally for students who cannot attend a workshop. Although it would seem that this wouldn't work as well, a distant attunement is just as powerful. I arrange a time with my student and have them sit in meditation while I perform the attunement from a distance. It can also be passed through a video. The student may have all the same sensations during and in the days following as if they received an in-person attunement. Of course, if you receive a distant attunement and then get the opportunity later to have one in person, you can always do another attunement at the same level.

Experiences during an attunement

What a student experiences during an attunement is similar to that of a recipient during a Reiki session but stronger. Although some students will feel nothing, the majority of students will feel or experience their attunement.

Physical Sensations – You may feel heat, cold, or tingling sensations. For example, you may feel a muscle twitch or you may sweat.

Dizziness – Occasionally students feel slightly dizzy. If this happens, just relax and your Reiki Master may instruct you to visualize tree roots of white light going down into Mother Earth to ground you.

Emotionally Overwhelmed – the Reiki energy may bring up and resolve issues within you as it clears your chakras. You may even see a glimpse of a past life or your soul purpose. It may also be a very happy emotion that makes you want to cry. Emotions are good. Allow yourself to release.

Laughing or Crying – You may experience uncontrollable giggling, laughter, or may even want to cry. Just accept and allow yourself to feel what ever you are experiencing.

Seeing Colors – Some sense bright lights or balls of light. This is simply the Reiki energy coming into you and your clairvoyant sense powering up. You may even see visions or receive messages.

Seeing Spirits – Some may see their guides or Reiki Masters in spirit. Students may even see Dr. Usui during an attunement.

After an Attunement

Immediately following any Reiki attunement there is a period where the cleansing can be intense. This often coincides with the 21 days of self-healing. Your guides continue to clear your chakras and align your energy during this period. If you had blockages (physical or spiritual), your Reiki guides will remove these blockages first. As your chakras are cleansed and aligned, anything that you didn't deal with may surface. This is a good thing as you are finally resolving and releasing negative energies that may have been causing you issues for years.

Cleansing takes place on all levels – physical, mental, emotional, and spiritual. The more the Reiki energy is allowed to flow, the more beneficial this will be. During this time, go easy on yourself and allow the process. Drink lots of water as this will help you to release toxins and flush out any negative energy that has surfaced. Your self-healing sessions will help you to release and cleanse more quickly. Take time to meditate daily. Allow yourself lots of sleep and rest. Taking walks in nature is very healing and may help you through this process.

Most students report some moments of emotion during this time. They usually report feeling wonderful, more energetic, healthy, and alive.

Preparation Before an Attunement

Some preparation the week before will help you to get the strongest connection out of your attunement. However, even if you don't do any preparation, you will still receive the energies, become a Reiki channel, and receive your Reiki Level One certificate. Your Reiki powers will also continue to enhance long after the class. These suggestions are not something to stress over, but if you have the time they may help strengthen your initial experience and minimize any negative feelings afterwards.

I usually send my students an email with notes to prepare for the class. Here are some preparation guidelines to help you get the most out of your attunement. Basically they are meant to clear your body and soul, and help you to get to your peak psychic acceptance.

Preparation for an Attunement

Limit or cut out animal protein for the 3 days prior. Fish is fine. This is to clear any negative energies from food.

If you have ever fasted and enjoy this process, fasting on juice or water beforehand is good. (1-2 days or just a few hours). If you are not used to this then just try to eat healthy.

Limit or stop any caffeinated drinks for 3 days.

Limit or no alcohol for 3 days.

Limit or no sugar or junk food for 3 days.

Limit or stop smoking cigarettes for 3 days.

Quiet negative outside distractions, news, horror movies, etc. for 3 days.

Try to spend some time appreciating nature each day.

Start as soon as possible and meditate daily, an hour if possible. If you are not able to meditate, just sit quietly and contemplate. Ask to release anger, fear, worry, and other negative feelings. Then spend some time contemplating or meditating on why you want to receive a Reiki attunement and what you wish to receive from your Reiki attunement. (e.g. to increase your psychic ability or to be able to heal yourself and others, mentally and physically, etc.)

If you use other rituals or methods to get your psychic powers stimulated, go ahead and start to prepare yourself. (e.g. crystals)

Again, many people do nothing beforehand, so don't stress about this, but a quiet contemplating period before would be good and at least avoid a heavy party weekend!

Chapter 10.
Colors of Chakra

Learn more about the colors of the chakras with our Color Chart of 7 chakras! Let's discuss the chakra symbols and how to energize the colors of the chakra through meditation, color breathing, chakra stones, clothing, decoration, and food!

Summary

The meaning of the colors of the chakra about Chakra color chart

We have seven major chakras or energy centers in the body, each with different functions and attributes. There are also seven chakra colors assigned to the chakras, each with its definition. What are the colors of the chakras? The colors of the chakra are red, orange, yellow, green, blue, indigo, and purple. The chakra color table below will give you a quick overview of what each of them means.

The colors of the chakras

Now let us know more about each of the seven colors and symbols of the chakra (see images). You have to learn more about the colors of the chakras and their functions; this can help you understand which part of you may need healing.

Color of the root chakra

The color of the root chakra is red and is connected to the adrenal glands. The associated body parts include the hips and legs, and the organs related to this chakra are the bladder and kidneys. Red is the most profound and lowest frequency of the color spectrum of the chakra. On an emotional level, red is identified as the color of passion, anger, and rage, danger or red alert, warmth, and energy. For example, when a person exercises or exercises himself, his cheeks often turn red due to excess heat and blood flow. Usually, those who identify with these emotions and wear red are people strongly linked to their physical form - and, as mentioned above - often neglect other elements of their nature, such as their emotional side and spiritual.

The root of chakra and the color red are also linked to the automatic fight or flight response when people feel in danger. This answer comes from a time when humans needed to defend themselves and protect themselves from damage such as predatory animals. This response served well as protection by injecting large doses of adrenaline and cortisol into the body, thus allowing bursts of energy to run or fight if necessary, hence the name "fight or flight." "Today, for most people, this danger no longer exists, and the answer is somewhat out of date. However, it is still active and can wreak havoc on the body. When you are stressed at work or watching an exciting movie, the fight or flight response can become aggressive.

When the root chakra is balanced and works in harmony, the energy becomes more robust. Emotions such as anger and automatic responses, such as struggle or flight, are less active. A result is a person who is better able to relax, who is not in control of his emotions, and who feels at peace.

Color of the sacred chakra

The color of the holy chakra is orange and is closely related to red in frequency but works at a maximum vibration.

The color of the sun and heat is Orange; He is expressive and creative and exudes energy and strength. The associated glands include the ovaries and testes, and the organs related to this chakra include the reproductive system and lower intestines.

Emotionally, orange identifies with happiness, vitality, joy, wisdom, and creativity. It is also associated with instinct. Connecting and feeding the energy of this chakra through the chakra of the solar plexus to the heart chakra allows the interaction of gut feelings with heart-based desires. This is important because most people act on a mental level of thought, ignoring the wisdom of their instincts and the direction of their hearts. This is the reason so many people feel lost and isolated. When the orange energy of the sacred chakra flows, it allows creative ideas to emerge, clear direction, and the achievement of life's purpose.

Color of the solar plexus chakra

Yellow is the color of the solar plexus chakra and, while maintaining the warm tones of red and orange, the lighter light of yellow brings clarity, knowledge, and power. Physically, the yellow color of the solar relates to the pancreas, digestive system, lower back, and muscles.

Emotionally, yellow evokes good humor, confidence, and positive self-esteem. When the energy of this chakra is blocked or stagnated, negative traits such as pessimism, competitiveness, selfishness, and feeling unworthy come. The solar plexus is the junction between the lower chakras, and the higher emotional and spiritual chakras, blockages in this chakra can lead to a disconnection between physical and mental nature. Excessive dependence on the lower chakras or overuse of the upper chakras leads to a feeling of disconnection and an inability to be fully present in the present.

Color of the heart chakra

The predominant color of the heart chakra is green, also associated with the color pink.

Green is the color of vitality, nature, growth and balance, while pink is the color of love, joy, new beginnings, and serenity. The two colors, while operating at different densities, work in harmony to create a balanced and liking heart chakra.

The physical parts of the heart chakra include the thymus, heart, lungs, shoulders, arms, and chest. On an emotional level, a balanced and fluid heart chakra promotes feelings of love, peace, happiness, empathy, and compassion. When the energy in this area weakens or becomes blocked, feelings of jealousy, resentment, lack, and loneliness can arise. The green color and the pink association of the heart chakra when they flow freely open the door to divine light and love.

Throat Chakra Color

The color of the throat chakra is a magnificent shade of turquoise blue. Blue means sky, openness for good things, fresh air, and liberation. The physical parts of the throat chakra are the thyroid gland, neck, throat, and ears. When operating in harmony, the desires of the heart are expressed and expressed through an open-throat chakra, while the intuitive third eye prompts are fed from the throat to an open and welcoming spirit, then conveyed through the throat. In this way, the sincere desires of an individual can be reflected and put into practice through their thoughts, actions. The throat chakra is best recognized for communication, spiritual role of this chakra is a divine expression and being true to yourself.

Color of the third eye chakra

A deep shade of indigo represents the color of the third eye chakra. However, the purple color is also associated with this chakra. The indigo and violet colors reflect mystery, wisdom, knowledge, prosperity, and spirituality. On the physical level, the third eye relates to the pituitary gland, eyes, sinuses, and brain. This chakra is the seat of inner knowledge or intuition, understanding - both spiritual and practical understanding, and connection - internal connection and connection with the whole. An unbalanced third eye chakra reveals stubbornness, self-esteem, pride, excessive self-confidence, and disconnect of emotional and another knowledge.

Crown Chakra Color

Crown chakra is purple in or, in some cases, pure white. Violet links the physical to the spiritual; this is equivalent to wisdom and divine power. White reflects the purity of spirit, the brilliance of pure light, and clarity. It is often one of the last chakras to open or activate completely. It remains dormant in many who operate only from their lower chakras and identify themselves only with the material world. When it is accessed, the crown chakra brings transformation, belonging, connection to the whole, and liberates from the concept of duality. From a physical point of view, the coronal chakra is linked to the pineal gland, the cerebral cortex, and the brain. The gifts that an open and functional crown chakra offers include the feeling of unity, peace, and being full or complete.

The seven chakras - Colors of the rainbow!

As described above, the primary colors associated with chakras include red, orange, yellow, green, blue, indigo, and purple. This means that the seven colors of the chakra are the same as the seven colors of the rainbow! For those who can see the atmosphere, it is as beautiful as the rainbow. The beauty of the rainbow that crosses the sky has been evoked and written over the centuries.

"Gratitude is the real treasure that God wants us to find because it is not the pot of gold but the rainbow that colors our world." - Richelle E. Goodrich

Why does the beauty of the rainbow resonate with those who stop to look at it? There is something about the beauty of the colors that are reflected in each person. A person who appreciates the colors of the rainbow appreciates its beauty. The magic of the fleeting vision of the spectrum of colors temporarily suspended in the sky deserves to be valued. This is reflected in the color spectrum of the chakra that each person holds. Everyone carries with them the colors of the rainbow, residing at a microscopic level in their energy field. In a sense, each person aspires to see what they know to be accurate, the beauty of the colors that make up their being. If each individual could see the rainbow in the colors of the chakra when they met, would they then treat themselves differently?

As with the rainbow, the color of the first chakra - the primary chakra - is red, followed by the orange of the sacred chakra and the yellow of the chakra of the solar plexus. These first three chakra colors constitute the lowest tones or color frequencies. Red, orange, and yellow evoke nature and autumn when the leaves change color. Meanwhile, even if life is preparing for sleep, the beauty of the changing colors is magnificent.

In this way, the colors of the lower chakra reflect the connection with nature, the grounding energy of Mother Earth, and the power and wisdom that lies within.

The colors of the upper chakra represent the waves of the lighter shade of green and pink in the heart chakra, blue in the throat chakra, indigo or purple in the third eye, and finally purple or white in the crown chakra. These lighter colors evoke thoughts of blossoming leaves and flowers, new beginnings, healing, expression, awareness, and feelings of love, joy, peace, and vitality.

How to invigorate the colors of the chakra!

After taking a closer look at the seven chakra colors and their meanings, it's time to find out how to take care of and nurture the positive aspects of the chakras and the energy system as a whole. Chakra color therapy helps to re-adapt and realign the chakras to their optimal frequency and to restore their function and balance. As mentioned earlier, each of the colors of the chakras operates on different frequencies. If the chakra is blocked or misaligned, the rate of colors also changes, often becoming slower and thus attenuating the intensity and vibrations of the energy center. To restore the frequency of colors and, therefore, the energy of the chakra, the use of the color chart of the chakra and chromotherapy can bring considerable advantages. Chroma chakra can be used through meditation, chromatic breathing,

These crystals vibrate at specific frequencies, and using the crystal colors associated with the chakras is a very effective way to cleanse and activate the chakras. Chakra stones are readily available for purchase and can be used at home or by therapists during healing or energy massage sessions. The use of crystals, in conjunction with energy healing, such as Reiki, can complement and improve treatment.

Meditation

Using a color during meditation is as simple as seeing the colors of the chakra in the energy field, for example, focusing on a specific color and seeing it envelop the body. Whatever color comes to mind, it is usually the color that best suits the individual and meets their basic needs at that time. The required color can change from day to day and even from minute to minute, depending on the mood, environment, and mental state.

Color Breath

It is a very effective way to revitalize and balance the chakras. The color of the chakras is considered to be breathed into the body by inspiration and releasing all gray and dark shades and energy during expiration.

Starting with red at the root chakra in the appropriate colors in each of the seven main chakras successively until you reach the crown chakra.

Food

It is known that root vegetables like potatoes, carrots, and beets, when eaten, help to anchor the chakras and the energy system.

It is not surprising that some of these root vegetables also syndicate the colors of the lower chakras. The colors of the food consumed not only provide nutrients to the body but also serve to improve the function of the chakras. It is, therefore, essential to eat and drink a wide variety of natural fruits and vegetables of different colors. However, the consumption of artificial colors, such as coloring added to processed foods, does not serve the same purpose and can hurt energy levels and health.

Clothing and decoration

Wearing specific colors is known to improve mood and attitude. However, the opposite may also be exact; for example, if a person has an overactive root chakra and tends to wear red, this can make the problem worse. Clothing colors can be used to harmonize and improve the chakras, but too much of one color can be too forceful. Likewise, the colors of the chakra system can be used at home and integrated into particular rooms to improve the desired ambiance in this area. Subtle shades of purple and blue can be used in bedrooms to create a soothing atmosphere, while more vibrant colors like orange and red can be added in moderation to living spaces to warm and invigorate the room.

Chapter 11.
Kundalini Awakening

The word Kundalini translates from Sanskrit as "coiled up." This word describes the concept that energy is coiled up at the base of the spine of every person living on earth. It is often depicted as a snake or serpent who lies within the pelvic bowl. As this energy is awakened, the serpent power rises up through the body and all the chakras until it reaches the crown of the head. This coil of energy or snake is the Life-Force, the prana, the divine power that when awakened will lead to an unraveling process, allowing consciousness to shift and become elevated into pure, divine, creation–energy consciousness.

Kundalini yoga is the body practice associated with this energy. The practice of which, along with other meditations, energy, work, and lifestyle choices help the practitioner come into alignment with this divine energy. There are several different yoga practices, each with its own philosophy, mantra and spiritual expression, or goal. Many people work with Kundalini Yogis or Gurus to experience a safe, healing experience, but it can also occur without the presence of such a teacher.

Exact origins of kundalini and the yoga practice created to inspire awakening are unknown. Ancient texts called Vedas, which the philosophies of Kundalini are derived from, are as old as 1000 BCE, and possibly early. Within the schools of Hinduism, the Vedic, Tantric, and Shakti philosophies, as well as Pranayama are linked to the concept of Kundalini. The Upanishads, part of the Vedic texts, detail the idea and concept of Kundalini. The concept of Kundalini-yoga, however, was not identified in these texts until later, sometime in the 16th century.

There are multiple Indic and Hindu religious contexts that blend together to bring about the practice of Kundalini awakening. Shaktism is the concept of divine, goddess energy, while Tantra literally means "loom, weave, system." Pranayama translated is "extension of the Life-force". All of these schools of thought, collaborating together, in addition to other ancient philosophies and texts, compile to create Kundalini and the theory of awakening this divine consciousness.

Essentially, this ancient philosophy, practice, and belief come from a long line of Indic, Hindu and Yogic beliefs and ideas, all of which have been somewhat recently exposed to our Western culture. Surprisingly, these practices were actually forbidden for Yogis to teach outside of the Indian lineage and culture. However, in 1968, a yogi named Harbhajan Singh Khalsa traveled to the U.S. and was spiritually called to help Western culture find enlightenment. At the time of the late '60s, American youth were grasping for heightened consciousness through the use of psychoactive drugs. Yogi Bhajan had the vision to elevate American culture with his ancient, sacred knowledge and taught many future yogis and gurus who continue to spread this knowledge for the good of all man, and womankind.

Since its beginnings, Kundalini has had many practitioners and the tradition of the master/student relationship has always been a big part of the awakening process. Many argue that it can be too uncomfortable to walk the path of Awakening without a skilled master, guru, or yogi; however, many people come into this kind of enlightenment, this higher consciousness through their own practice and life experiences, although it can take longer, depending on circumstances and devotion to awakening. There are some key Gurus and Yogis to know of who have played important roles in the philosophy, practice, and teaching of Kundalini. Below are just a few to get you started.

Guru Nanak (1469-1539)

Author of Japji Sahib (The Song of the Soul), this book was his personal explanation of enlightenment based on his own unexpected enlightenment experience. According to his writings, he went to take a bath and when he was in the water, he stayed under the water for 3 days without surfacing. His meditation was so deep, and his breath so slow that he was able to maintain life for this long without coming up for air. Beneath the water, he envisioned the cosmic force of all that is, the infinite potential and power within us all that is pure creation and divine consciousness. When he surfaced, he wrote The Song of the Soul to share his discovery and teach enlightenment.

Swami Vivekananda (1863-1902)

This Hindu Monk is recognized for his introduction of the concept of Yoga and other Indian religious and spiritual practices to Western culture. Although it wasn't until the 1960s when Yogi Bhajan began to teach the practices, Swami Vivekananda brought awareness of the philosophies of Hinduism and Yoga to America in 1893 at the Parliament of the World's Religions. Notions of Hindu and Yoga practices were relatively unknown and Swami Vivekananda brought these concepts to the status of significant world religious practices.

Swami Nigamananda (1880-1935)

Associated with Shaktism, Tantra yoga and other Hindu practices, he is known for a type of yoga called laya-yoga. Laya is the Sanskrit word for "dissolve." According to this yogic practice, the dissolving of the self allows for the merging of Divine Consciousness, a major component in the foundations of Kundalini Awakening. Swami Nigamananda was adamant that Laya Yoga was different from Hatha Yoga in that Hatha promotes strength and vitality of the physical body, while Laya attains a connection to the Divine.

Swami Sivananda (1887-1963)

Founder of The Divine Life Society in 1936, physician, author and eventually, monk, Swami Sivananda penned hundreds of books on the topics of yoga, meditation, and enlightenment. It combined Laya Yoga principles, along with other Hindu and yogic sources outlining the path to awakening to source energy. His book accompanied the uprise in Western, Neo-Hindu practices in the late 1960s that contributed to the Enlightenment counterculture.

B.K.S. Iyengar (1918-2014)

Considered the "father of modern yoga" by many, B.K.S. Iyengar is the creator of Iyengar yoga and was one of the world's leading yoga teachers. He wrote many books on the subject of yoga and was one of a handful of Yogis who popularized yoga practices in today's world. His oldest daughter, Geeta Iyengar (1944-2018), was notable in the promotion of yoga for women's health.

The organization is a massive resource of education, community and lifestyle practices that allows the brilliance of the soul to glow in every aspect of life. From what you eat, how you dress, how you speak, how you experience relationships, how you teach and raise your kids, how you run your business, Yogi Bhajan brought all the concepts of Kundalini into the teachings of his organization to aid in the transformation of the collective human consciousness. The organization's principles are also largely based in Sikh Dharma which is what Guru Nanak founded in the 15th century, promoting unity consciousness for the good of all humankind.

Chapter 12.
How To Awaken The Kundalini

Now that you have some background and history about what Kundalini is and where it comes from, you may wonder, why awaken this energy? Why not practice other forms of yoga and meditation that will help you feel in alignment and at peace with life?

Kundalini Awakening can be very intense and the experience of ascension is different for everyone. It can turn your whole world and life upside-down. You may change your whole lifestyle, or fearlessly start your dream job; you may move to another country to practice your new wholeness and enlightenment in a like-minded community, and you may become a benefactor or a volunteer. Sometimes it can be scary and unpredictable to begin such a journey. It's easy to keep things the way they are, but if you know that you have the power within you to awaken your divine energy, your higher consciousness, and ultimately the source of your primal spark, the energy of creation, why wouldn't you?

There are so many significant benefits to taking this path

of transformation for your mind, body, and spirit. Below are some of the advantages of an awakened existence through the process of Kundalini Awakening.

Mind

Overall enhancement of memory and cognitive ability; clear thinking.

Ability to face the uncontrollable and unpredictable ups and downs of life with more peace and tranquility.

Greater mental focus and self-control.

Enhanced senses and perceptions.

Reduction in feelings of anger, shame, guilt, depression, and anxiety.

Self-love and compassion and empathy for others.

Increased or awakened psychic capabilities.

Body

More balanced and healthy function of various body systems including digestion, lymphatic flow, and cardiovascular health.

Stronger and more balanced immune system.

Elimination of bad habits such as smoking, excessive alcohol or drug use, and over-eating.

Overall improvement in physical strength.

Increase in energy and vitality.

Can possibly eradicate ongoing or chronic health issues such as irritable bowel syndrome, kidney stones, edema, and skin discoloration due to poor circulation.

Better sleep.

Spirit

Increase in a spiritual connection with self, others, and the Universe.

Higher vibrational frequency in your body's energy to magnetically attract things, situations, and people to you with your thoughts.

Heightened awareness of the flows of energy in all life and matter.

Balanced chakras and inner energies that lead to an overall feeling of alignment and transcendence.

Awakened inner-eye or third eye to promote connection to the divine, experience visions, astral travel, and latent psychic abilities.

Spiritual radiance, bliss, peace, healing, and calm.

These are several of the benefits and of course, there are more. Kundalini awakening is such a gift to the soul, to the individual consciousness and to the realization that we are all connected and have this special opportunity to become more enlightened, evolved, healed, and in tune to our greatest gift of Divine consciousness. The benefits of transformation, enlightenment, and transcendence far outweigh costs. And what is the cost, you may ask. The cost, dear reader, is that you commit yourself to an amazing journey of self-discovery, a path of inner enrichment and an embodiment of feeling one with the Universe.

The awakening of the Kundalini has been linked to various health benefits. It promotes good health at many levels. It regulates and corrects blood pressure; it is also an effective stress reliever; it can fight and even cure diabetes and other diseases, as well as a host of many other physical benefits. This also involves relief from stomach and liver problems, even issues with kidney stones and gallstones. There are even those who claim that awakening the Kundalini can cure serious diseases like cancer. Indeed, when you experience the power that surges through your body upon awakening of the Kundalini, you will know that indeed, everything is possible. Having clarity of thought is a very common benefit of awakening the Kundalini, as well as increased focus, attention, and mental power.

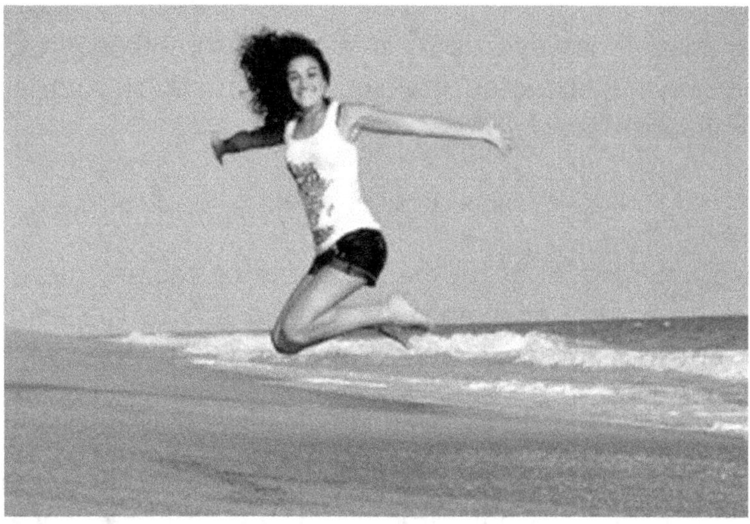

It is also worth noting that many of these benefits can be enjoyed even without fully awakening your Kundalini. The different practices themselves, as you will learn from this book, can give you tons of health benefits. Of course, if you want to experience the benefits to their fullest potential, then you need to actually awaken your Kundalini.

Different Kundalini exercises and meditations

It should be noted that there is no single exercise or meditation technique that will guarantee the awakening of the Kundalini. The accumulative spiritual practices and spiritual maturity are needed for this to happen. All the practices in this book will help you awaken your Kundalini. However, be reminded that gaining knowledge is not enough. You also need to put that knowledge into actual and continuous practice.

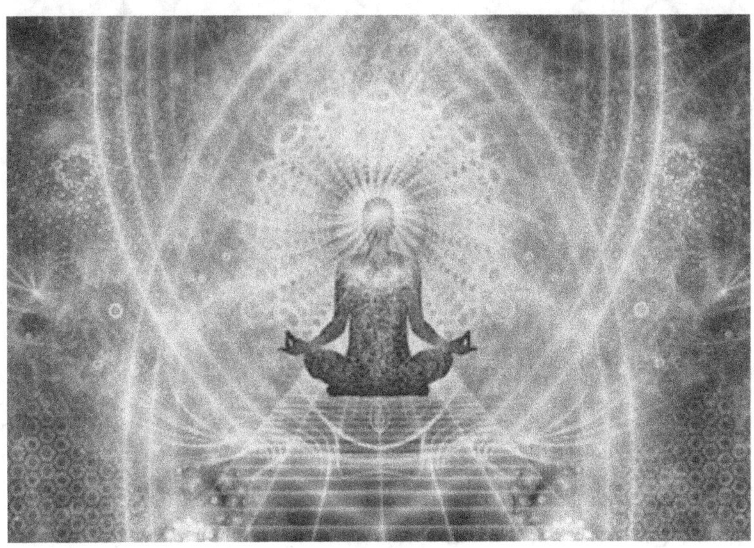

You may wonder why this book is full of mental and meditative techniques. The reason is that the awakening the Kundalini is more of a mental effort and practice. You should expect to engage in long hours of meditation. However, there are also physical exercises that can help you awaken the Kundalini. After all, physical exercises of any kind are a natural way of cleansing the body of negative energies. Depending on your physical fitness, you may engage in a physical activity or exercise of your choice. For starters, you might want to engage in some walking exercises. If you are a feeling fit and healthy, then you can go for a jog or a good run. Needless to say, exercising is also good for the physical body.

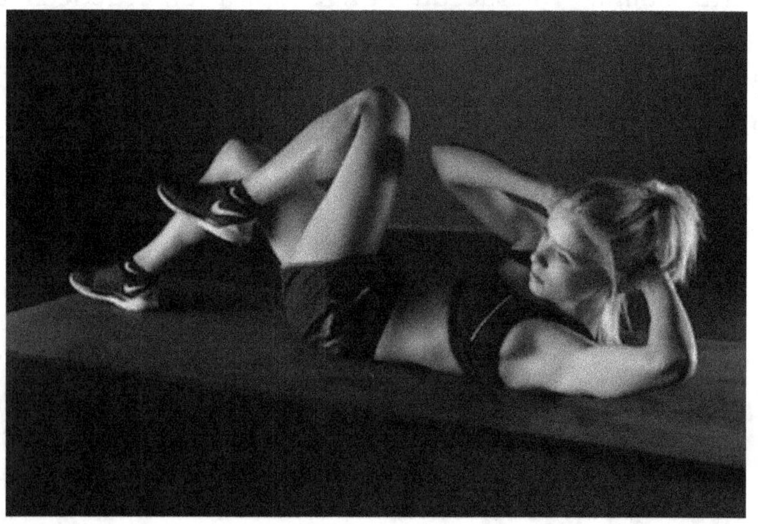

The best way to awaken the Kundalini is by doing meditation. As you read this book, you will learn different meditation techniques. Some of these meditation techniques will directly empower and engage your Kundalini, while others may do so indirectly. Still, it is worth noting that all meditation practices help in awakening the Kundalini. Hence, you can rest for sure that no effort will ever be wasted.

The effects of Kundalini activation on the body, emotions, and the mind

As to the emotions, it will make you feel more centered and calm. In fact, even before you reach the stage of awakening, you will already enjoy its positive effects on the emotional level.

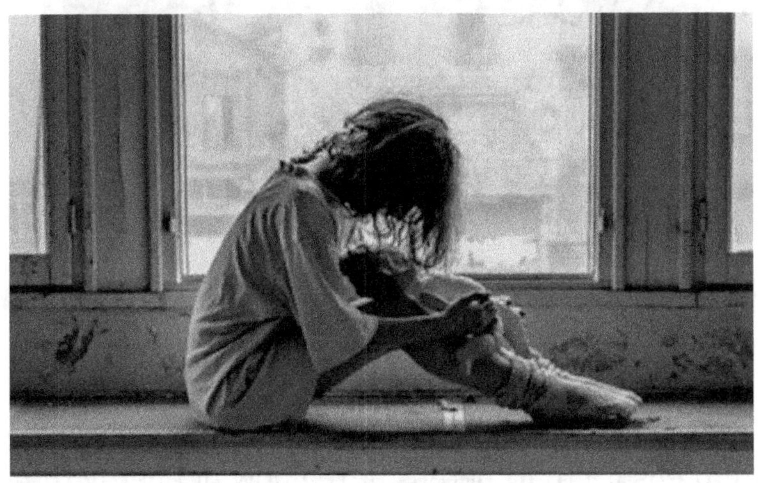

With regard to the mind, you will have more mental clarity. You will be able to think and analyze things more clearly. It will give you such clarity that you have never experienced in your life. In fact, it is with such mental clarity that is tantamount to having complete peace of mind.

How Kundalini feels

If your Kundalini is still dormant, then you might not feel it at all. However, the more that you work on your Kundalini, the more that you can feel it, especially when you do the meditation techniques that directly engage the Kundalini. At the moment of the awakening of the Kundalini, you can expect for a powerful rush of energy through your body.

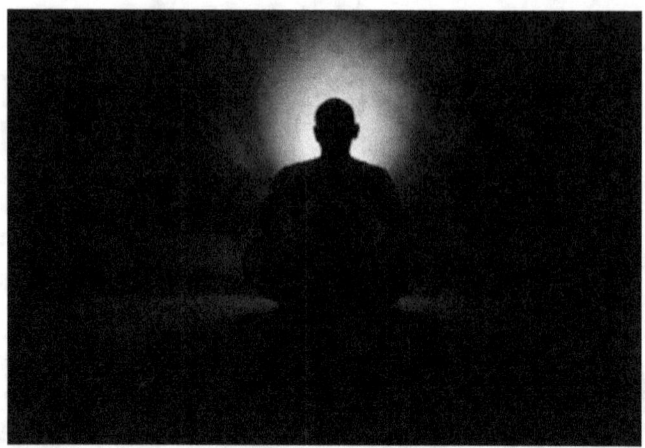

How to clear the blockages that prevent Kundalini from rising smoothly

Blockages can prevent the awakening and rising of the Kundalini. In order to avoid this from happening, you need to ensure that there is a free flow of energy through the energy channels meridians. You should also ensure that your chakras are cleansed and aligned. Do not worry; you will learn how to do this later in the book.

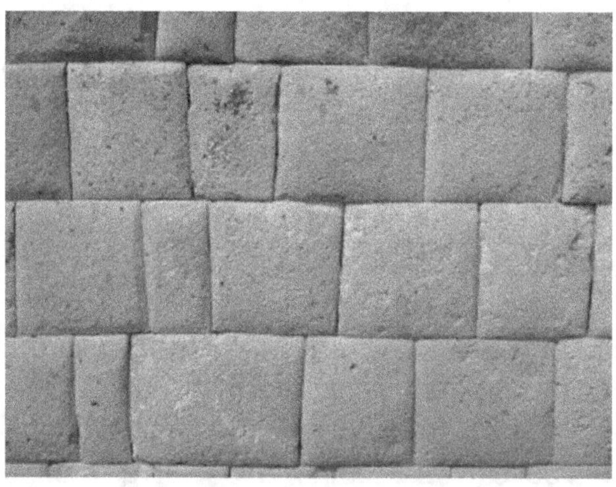

However, what causes these blockages? There are many causes of blockages. A common cause of this is having too much stress. In the modern world, being stressed has become very common; and this is actually a sad thing, as it means that many people do not enjoy a free flow of energy. If you want to activate your Kundalini, then you need to be sure to manage your stress levels effectively. It should be noted that stress itself is not bad; it is when you fail to manage it properly that it becomes bad for you. There are many other causes that can impede the free flow of energy, such as having bad experiences, emotional breakdown, psychic attacks, and others. When treating blockages, it is important to note the reason or the main cause of the problem. A common mistake is to treat a blockage without attending to what causes it in the first place. Therefore, if a blockage is due to your stress at work, then you need to make some adjustments at work. You cannot just treat the effect or the result without going after the source.

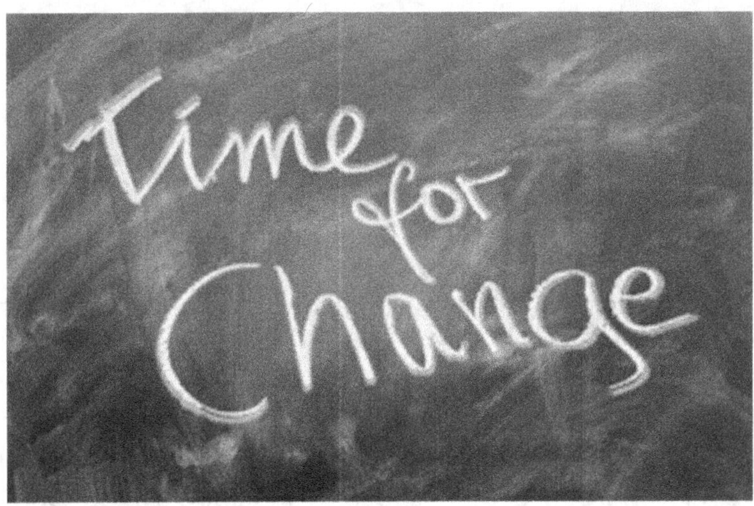

Therefore, removing of any blockages or healing should

be done on two levels, physical and spiritual. On the physical level, you may have to make some lifestyle changes.

How to awaken a dormant Kundalini

As already mentioned, there is no single rule or practice that can guarantee the awakening of the Kundalini. This will have to depend on your overall spiritual maturity and practices. However, generally, there are two ways to awaken a dormant Kundalini: by yourself or with the help of a spiritual master.

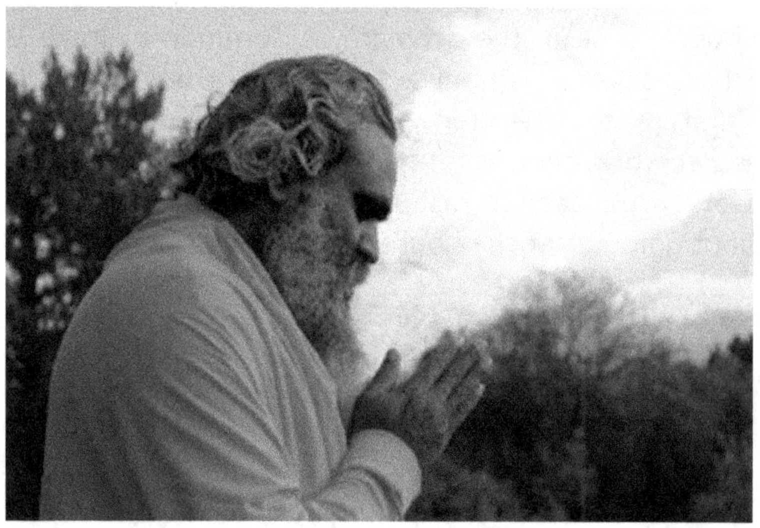

Being able to do it on your own is exactly what this book is about. However, if you want to do it with the help of a spiritual master or guru, then this would involve complete dedication and submission to your master. Your master may also require you to do certain meditation practices; however, there are also those who claim to be able to awaken one's Kundalini as long as the disciple relinquishes everything and submits to his/her master.

The problem here is that it is not easy to find a real master. Unfortunately, there are so many people out there who claim to be a master but are, in reality, just merely full of hacks and shams. Another problem with this approach is that although a master may be able to awaken your Kundalini, your soul might not be ready for it. This refers to your spiritual maturity. Therefore, when it comes to awakening the Kundalini, it is strongly advised that you do the work yourself so that your soul can mature and make you be ready for it. Of course, you are still free to ask help from a master but do not neglect your own spiritual growth.

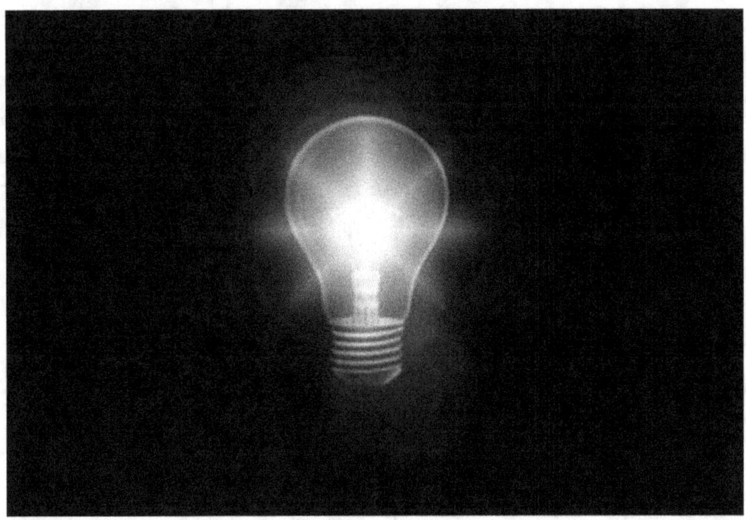

It is probably safe to assume that your Kundalini lies dormant in our right now, which explains why you are reading this book. Do not worry, as this book will guide you and teach you the techniques that will allow you to awaken the serpentine power. Just stay with me so you can gain knowledge as you follow me on this journey of true Kundalini awakening.

Chapter 13.
Tips For Daily Practice

Both practitioners and recipients of Reiki treatment have to ensure that they are well versed with what Reiki is and the right way to provide or receive it. It is not simply about channeling the energy but rather making sure that the energy does the work intended and achieves the expected benefits. Therefore, learning alone and even acquiring the status of a master is not enough if the process is not done per the guidelines that have been handed over the years to the present day. Other guidelines might not, however, be traditional ones but are just meant to make sure that your sessions are peaceful.

You can connect to the energy fields but what happens after connecting and once you are done with the session. These are some of the things that, if you consider, will help you move from just being an average Reiki practitioner to an excellent performer. Most importantly, your sessions will be more productive. Remember that it is not what so much what you know that determines what you get but rather how you do it. With that in mind, here are some of the very vital general guidelines that you ought to remember and put into practice whenever preparing for, during, and after Reiki sessions.

Take Deep Centering Breaths before Session

Every time you get ready to start a Reiki session, take some time to take centering breaths as a way of putting your body in the right state of action. Breaths often bring a relaxing feeling and also put your mind in a meditating mood. With such a state of mind, it is easy to proceed consciously aware of what is happening around you.

Another very centering thing to do as you get ready to start your Reiki session is to hold your hands and say a prayer that expresses your wish. While praying, visualize yourself having what you are praying for and try to connect to the field of love that is inside you. Take a few minutes and do it slowly, so you create the best atmosphere for the forthcoming healing session.

Combining a prayerful or meditative mind with deep belly breaths is already the first step to healing, and when you start the Reiki session, it won't take long before you get the healing effect that you desire. All these activities are not meant to decorate the process but to prepare you well in readiness for your Reiki healing session.

Understand Your Reiki Practice Level and Enhance It

As already explained in this book, there are three levels of Reiki, namely the first-degree level, second degree, and the third/master level. Each level is effective, and anyone practicing Reiki at any level should not feel inferior or superior to anyone else because of the state that they are in or have attained. The most important thing is to make all your sessions effective by allowing energy to flow in yourself freely.

If you are at the beginner's level, start your sessions with a spiritual affirmation and make simple intents each time. Starting with a positive intent will always make it easy for you to go through all your sessions. For those at the second-degree level or distance healing, always make sure that the symbols you use to represent your subject are the correct ones bearing the right information or the right Reiki sequence. You are free to pick the symbols, but make sure that whichever you pick is what will help you achieve the desired outcome. For master, let your sessions or teachings to new beginners promote good Reiki practice.

Observe Touch Etiquette

Reiki involves touch as a way of channeling energy from the practitioner to the receiver or patient. For effectiveness and as a precaution it's always good to observe touch etiquette and seek the permission of the client first before you do it. Some might not be comfortable being touched; hence you wouldn't be right as a practitioner to go ahead and assume that everyone is comfortable with touch during Reiki.

Also, as a reminder, since this is explored in couple Reiki, some touch activities during the session are only permitted under spouses or life-partners settings. That should thus guide your practice, especially if you are a Reiki practitioner offering it to clients or patients in need of it. In some instances, touch might not be necessary, especially when it is distance Reiki. Whichever way, the right touch etiquette ought to be observed at all times for peaceful and not offensive session or healing moments.

Explain Reiki to Patients First If You are a Practitioner

Talk to your clients first and make it clear what Reiki is and what it is not before you go ahead to start your sessions with them. Let them know that Reiki is universal energy and that your role as the practitioner is to channel the energy to them to allow relaxation and healing. It is a healing process and does not use any drugs or invasive methods commonly used in medical healthcare provision centers.

Explaining the process also lets your clients be aware of or know what to expect during the session. Remember that some of them might want to take up the practice so that they will always be doing it on themselves. Nothing should, therefore, be hidden or unclear to the patient or recipient of Reiki healing. So always clear the air as a way of creating the right atmosphere for the natural healing process to take place.

A Quiet Place Is the Best for Reiki

Although Reiki can be done anywhere, masters or those who've practiced for years will tell you that a quiet environment is the best. Such a place promotes relaxation, a condition that is necessary, or a requirement for healing. If you can get a free quiet room at home for use every day as you practice Reiki, then your sessions will be effective. Balancing your body is essential, and doing so in a quiet room is easy compared to a place where there are possible distractions once you start the practice.

Reiki provides physical, mental, emotional as well as spiritual healing. Some of these can only be done in a quiet environment. You cannot, for instance, promote emotional or spiritual healing in a noisy place. Therefore, any kind of distraction, whether it is in the form of pictures, congestion, or simply not quiet, can affect the productivity of your sessions. That's, of course, not what you want; hence it is to make sure that you get the right place that will work well and promote peaceful Reiki sessions.

Other practices like consistency, continuously learning how Reiki works, and sharing experiences with like-minded Reiki enthusiasts can help make your sessions highly effective. Many people practice Reiki because they have heard how it works and the possible benefits that it brings to those who are good at it. However, how you carry it out is what determines the kind of results you will achieve at the end. It is not about just doing it or seeking the help of a good practitioner, but it is rather about understanding how it works. Learning should, therefore, be one of your ways of getting more information about Reiki and how you can use it for your good. Indeed, it is a unique healing process, and it is hard to understand it if you compare it to what happens in hospitals since its healing modalities are different.

Ethical Principles for Professional Reiki Practitioners

In some countries where Reiki has been taken and even incorporated into healthcare, there are ethical principles that practitioners should observe every time they are offering Reiki healing services to patients. Knowing that such principles exist is great, especially for learners who might want to practice in the future. They affect many areas of practice and dictate what can be done and what should be avoided from initial contact to when the session ends.

Reiki Contracts

- ❖ A practitioner should explain fully either in writing or verbally all the activities involved and procedures to the client before commencing the healing session.

- ❖ A practitioner should not advertise Reiki as a cure since that is a term used in the medical field or where there are invasive procedures

- ❖ Anything additional to the therapy should be permitted by the client first before it is done

- ❖ A declaration should be made on whether the treatment is offered freely and voluntarily or is to be paid for by the client

- ❖ Licensing, certificates, and qualifications of the Reiki practitioner must be displayed

Confidentiality

- ❖ All information provided by the client before the session as their concerns or intentions should be kept confidential, and the practitioner should never disclose to anyone unless with the consent of the client.

- ❖ For practitioners who work as a group or transfer their interest should never transfer the client's information without their permission to a new practitioner.

❖ If the client suffers from any serious condition, and they disclose it to the practitioner or provide medical records, the information provided should be protected and never disclosed without their permission.

Records

❖ Professional Reiki practitioners ought to keep clear records indicating when the sessions were carried out, time spent, and the number of sessions. Dates are very important and should be captured accurately.

❖ Information provided should be kept safely for up to seven years from the last session

❖ If the client dies for any reason even including those not related to Reiki and was an active member or regularly attending healing sessions, the practitioner should find correct ways of disposing of the records

❖ A client should never be forced to provide any information that might not be necessary or relevant for Reiki healing purposes

Soliciting Clients

❖ Professional Reiki clients should never practice client poaching habits from other professionals. Clients should come voluntarily based on the services provided and the general performance of the practitioner or quality of services provided.

The principles explained here apply only in some

countries such as the UK, but in other parts of the world, the practice is not governed by any law; hence it is practiced freely by those who believe in it. If you intend to become a practitioner, understanding these principles will help whether they are enforced or not in your area.

Chapter 14.
Conclusion Regarding Reiki

Again, the question, what is Reiki? Reiki is the universal energy flowing in and around us all. It is the life-giving energy available freely to anyone who seeks it out. Reiki is pure and lasts for the entirety of your life. It is a natural healing process.

Reiki is a gift from God, there are no fakes, no alternatives. It is one of a kind. No one person can claim rights to this wonderful energy. Anyone can learn and practice Reiki, there are no IQ requirements, no GPAs to be concerned about, no age, religious background, and no gender restraints. Reiki does not discriminate based on ethnicity or national origin. It is multi-national, multi-racial, world-wide, ever present, never ending energy coming straight from God or whomever you deem a higher power.

Reiki will change every part of your existence. It will heal the spiritual you, the emotional you. Reiki will help heal relationships, broken hearts, and stress levels.

Today throughout the world there are numerous Reiki organizations and practitioners. Each has developed their own ways of practicing Reiki. Each has their own tenets. Before choosing a Reiki Master to learn from, research to ensure he or she is practicing Reiki in the purest form possible. You will want to steer clear of imposters and people who have diluted the energy with other forms of holistic medicine or science.

When you find your medical treatment has not left you feeling fully healed you can turn to a complimentary treatment in Reiki to either speed recovery or assist in the reduction of pain associated with medical conditions or surgeries.

Whether you want to strengthen your resolve and firm up your spiritual aura or heal a sick relative, Reiki can be the wisest path.

We're finally at the end of the book. From the meaning to the techniques, you have learned what Reiki is and how it can be beneficial for you. It may have a bit of a tricky history and a mixed reception worldwide, especially with the many naysayers out there, but as you have learned, a lot of people think that it has allowed them to feel better and refreshed. Others can even say that the pain they once felt is gone because of it. They even get better sleep, too. And many have also integrated Reiki so well into their lives that they have ascended through the levels, got their attunements, and become practitioners themselves. Thus, they can share what they have learned with others.

Reiki has also been a great healing method. Even when the techniques are a bit challenging to do, they have turned into natural skills as time has passed by and revealed that energy can be cultivated with patience and perseverance. Even the simple act of meditation has become a growing trend in the world of Reiki.

Furthermore, Reiki healing is not just about the techniques themselves. It is also about fulfilling principles, being open to everyone, knowing that within ourselves is the energy we've all had right from the start, integrating the essence of the symbols that represent Reiki, and sharing what we have learned to everyone else who needs it.

After all, who would have thought that a rich doctor who went on a 21-day fast would envision the symbols that would build up the foundation for Reiki? With what Dr. Mikao Usui taught his students, his legacy for cultivating energy has lived on. Since then, it has touched many lives, built different types, branched out to everyone from all religions, and provided a new kind of light to millions of people.

Still, do not think that ascending to the highest Reiki level entails that your journey is over. No, it has only just begun. You will find the path towards learning more about Reiki and how it will benefit and bring you wonders that you have never thought possible in your life. It is also a way to see that Reiki has evolved.

Eventually, you may realize that Reiki is not just a healing method that you can learn and master: It can also be a lifestyle that will help you cultivate the energy you have waited for so long to have. It will be a way for you to carve a new path with opportunities and show you that you can control your fate.

You may not be able to control everything in life, but if you can channel the energy on the things you can, it will fill you up with the kind of light that you will never forget.

Reiki can show you that deep within your heart is a light that you can use to heal yourself and others.

So, what are you waiting for? Go for it, practice Reiki techniques, and feel the energy flow from within!

Chapter 15.
Introduction to Chakras

The history of the Chakras is one that is rich with different opinions and various origins. Many religious and spiritual belief systems contain information that relates to the Chakra system, but each has its own words, terminology, and overarching rules. What remains the same, however, is the basic understanding that contained within the body is a powerful energy that can have a wide range of effects on our mental, physical, and spiritual health.

Regardless of your own personal religious or spiritual background, the knowledge of the Chakras can have a positive impact on your own life, making it very worthwhile to take the time to understand. But before we dive into why the Chakras are so integral, we must first begin with what exactly they are.

The Meaning behind the Chakras

The word Chakra is derived from an Indian word "Chakra" which literally translates to mean "wheel". Each Chakra can be visualized as a spinning wheel within the body that houses the energy of that particular system. In total, there are seven distinct Chakras, each controlling and maintaining a certain part of the body, as well as different qualities within us. The Chakras are both located within the physical body, as well as being a mental and spiritual focal point for us to use within meditation and other energy healing rituals.

Many of us understand that the mind and bodywork in tandem, affecting one another and influencing how each functions. But, few of us truly understand the difference between the physical body and the mental energy that sounds it, and how those two systems are integral to one another. In all traditions that incorporate the knowledge of the Chakras, it is accepted that there is an energy that surrounds and runs through the body. This energy is commonly referred to as the "subtle body", a term that helps differentiate the physical experience from the spiritual one. The subtle body corresponds to a plane of existence that is outside of the physical realm in which we exist. This plane is connected to a higher concept, a higher realm of existence, and is spiritual rather than physical.

The concepts of the subtle body and various planes of existence can be extremely complicated and difficult to understand, so to avoid confusion we will focus just on the Chakras and how they impact the physical experience of all of us.

While we cannot actually see the Chakras, their influence in our lives can be felt daily. In total, there are seven different Chakras, which form a line from the foot of our spine up to the top of our head. Some religious belief systems disagree about how many Chakras there are, with some saying there are only five, and others saying there are thousands, but the most common understanding accepts the standard seven.

Each Chakra, as you can see, corresponds to a particular area of the body and it has a great impact on each of those systems. When the Chakras are closed off or unbalanced, they can result in physical ailments and other problems which can negatively impact our lives. In order to have a healthy and functioning mental and physical experience, it is encouraged that each person learns how to open each Chakra and keep them balanced and circulating.

Now, you may be asking yourself what exactly is meant when we talk about opening or balancing your Chakras. If you are struggling in your personal relationships, have difficulty sleeping, feel anxious, or get sick easily, then you may have an imbalance in your Chakras that are helping to cause these problems. If you can focus on each of the Chakras, you can identify where you are stuck and the underlying cause that is creating the imbalance. From here, through various exercises and techniques, you can fix the issue so that your energy flows properly once more.

Origins of the Chakra System

The Chakra system can be traced back many centuries, with the first usage of the term Chakras being seen in the Hindu Vedas. Written in ancient India, the Vedas are some of the oldest religious texts in existence and can be dated back to around the 1st and 2nd century BCE.

Chapter 16.
Identifying Chakras

'Chakra' is a Sanskrit word meaning wheel. The earliest recorded mention of the Chakras is at least 5000 years old. Hindu scriptures, called the 'Vedas,' have an elaborate description of the chakra system and the role it plays in our lives. The Buddhist and Jain scriptures also have the mention of the chakra system. Chakras are not a new discovery or gimmick. The power of chakras had been discovered thousands of years ago, and people made use of that knowledge to remain healthy and happy even when modern medical science was not at their disposal. Understanding of the chakras can help you in discovering some interesting things about health and life.

We all have a physical body that can be seen, touched, and felt. It consists of an elaborate system of blood, bones, muscles, nerves, and the works. However, besides the physical body, there is also an energy body. It consists of the energy that flows inside us. It keeps us powered and makes the system work.

Our body is a big bundle of energy. There is a constant energy transfer going on. Every part of the body needs energy. However, the needs of every part are different. All the body parts do not need energy at the same rate or quantity. The role of the chakras is to regulate this flow and ensure that you achieve your maximum potential.

The chakras are the energy centers. They are the points at which the concentration of this energy is at its peak. These chakras are constantly transferring energy to various parts of the body. The complete system of health and well-being relies heavily upon the functioning of these chakras. If the chakras work in tandem, you will remain healthy and joyful. They will have a profound impact on your physical, mental, emotional, and spiritual well-being.

The Vedas state that there are 144 major and minor chakras in our body. Out of these, there are two chakras that don't need your attention. The remaining 142 chakras play a very active role in ensuring your physical, mental, emotional, and spiritual health.

The chakras are strategically located at the junction points of our nervous system. They ensure a smooth transfer of energy.

These chakras are further divided into seven major chakras that would determine your personality, strengths, and weaknesses. Various factors related to your physical and mental health are also regulated by these chakras.

All seven major chakras are located along your spine. These chakras do not have a physical presence, as they are simply energy points. However, their location on your spine does have a significant impact on the organs in those areas. By keeping your chakras balanced, you can ensure that your vital organs keep working smoothly.

Chakras are constantly spinning energy wheels. Every chakra transfers energy to the other, and this process carries on until the seventh chakra. The higher you go up the chakra scale, the level of intensity it brings into your life would increase. It means if a lower chakra in your body is dominant, it will empower your abilities to feel the worldly pleasures more intensely. You will be able to enjoy the bounties of nature in a better way, as the lower three chakras relate to physical needs, whereas the upper three chakras cater to intellectual needs. If any of the upper three chakras is dominant in your body, you will have a greater affinity toward intellectual and spiritual realization. The higher the chakra, the greater will be the intensity with which it affects your life.

Each chakra has its important characteristics. Whichever chakra becomes dominant in you will give you its traits. It means that your personality is a very good reflection of the most powerful chakra in your body.

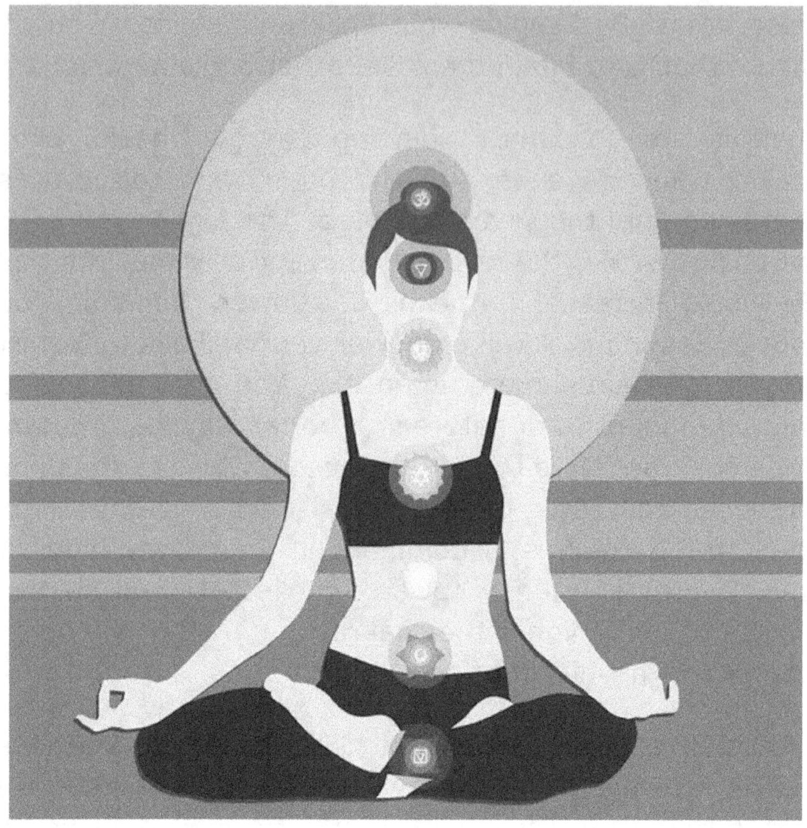

The seven main chakras in our body are the following.

The Root Chakra (Muladhara)

This is the first chakra in our body. It is located at the base of the spine. The most important role of this chakra is to provide you survival instincts. If this chakra is more powerful in your body, basic things like food and sleep will be the most important in your life. These two things may seem to be simple or trivial needs, but if you think deeply, the biggest part of our life revolves around only these two things. All the money we earn and the material wealth we gain is focused on survival and security. Food represents survival, and sleep represents security. This chakra keeps you centered in reality. You feel grounded and connected with basic human nature. Although this is the base chakra, it doesn't mean it is any less important. In fact, even if you seek the realization of the top chakra, proper functioning of the root chakra is of utmost importance. This is the chakra that will help you in remaining focused on reality while you strive for spiritual awakening.

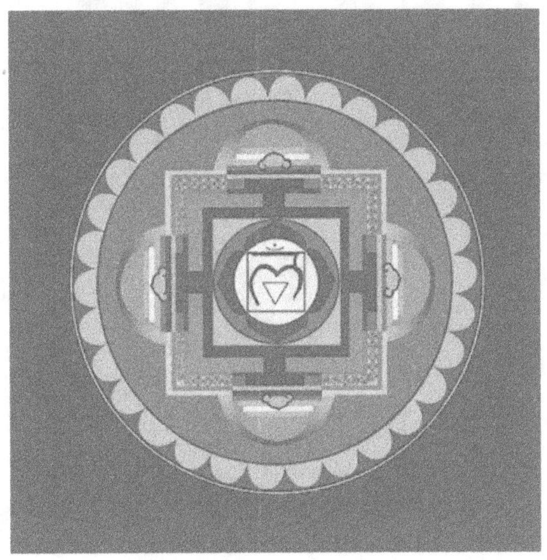

The Sacral Chakra (Svadishthana)

This is the pleasure seeker's chakra. Located approximately two inches below the navel, this chakra gives you the gift to enjoy this world. If this chakra becomes powerful in your body, you will be able to relish all the physical pleasures of this world. Most of the people in this world are unfortunate as they live in the most scenic places but never find them beautiful. Some people can cook the most tasteful delicacies but may not enjoy eating them. A person with power in this chakra will not be among them. A person with power in the sacral chakra will be able to enjoy even the most mundane activities in life. Such a person would have an eye to find joy even in the most inanimate objects. Power in this chakra enables you to live a joyful life. You wouldn't treat life as another passing affair as most of us do. For you, life will be a grand event, and you will have a big role in the grand scheme of things.

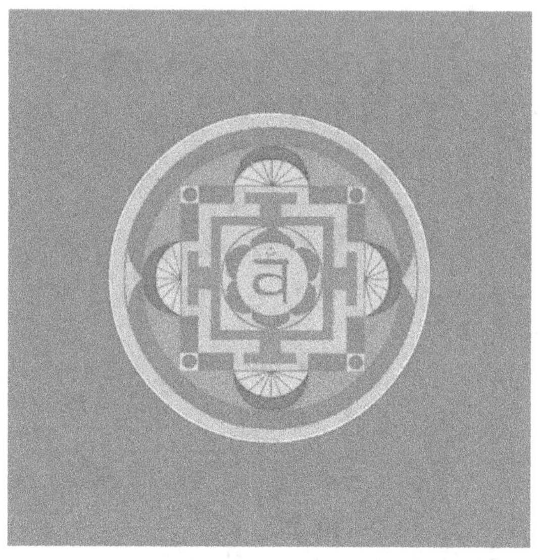

Solar Plexus Chakra (Manipura)

This is the doer's chakra, physically located around two inches above the navel. If this chakra finds expression in your body, it will give you indomitable will and the ability to make your dreams come true. It will make you enterprising. You will become a person who would enjoy working tirelessly. This chakra makes people efficient, hardworking, and zealous. Whether it is the field of politics, education, science, or commerce, this chakra can make you shine in every field. A person with this chakra in dominance would not understand the vice of procrastination. You'd never be able to leave work for tomorrow. 'If something can be done today, it must be done immediately' would be your life mantra. This chakra can make you intense and deeply focused.

The Heart Chakra (Anahata)

This chakra is located in the center of your chest. The meaning of this chakra is the unstruck sound, which means the energy of this chakra knows no bounds. It is boundless and ever-expanding. This is the center chakra in your body. Out of the seven chakras, this is the chakra that comes between the top and bottom three chakras. It is equidistant from the chakras that increase your attachment to the body and also from the chakras that increase your affinity toward intellectuality and spirituality. This is the chakra that helps you in finding a middle ground. It enables you to be creative. This means that you can find intellectual and spiritual meaning in the physical things of this world. This chakra can change the way you look at this world. It makes you more sensitive, emotional, generous, and empathetic. If this chakra is more powerful in your body, you will be able to feel the pain of the most impassive things in this world and express them with greater intensity. It makes you a creative person by nature. This is the fourth chakra in your body. Hence, the intensity of this chakra is higher than those preceding it. If it is a pain of others, you will be able to feel it very deeply. You may get disturbed when looking at others in pain. Tears may well up in your eyes whenever you deal with something emotional. You will live life much more intentionally than others.

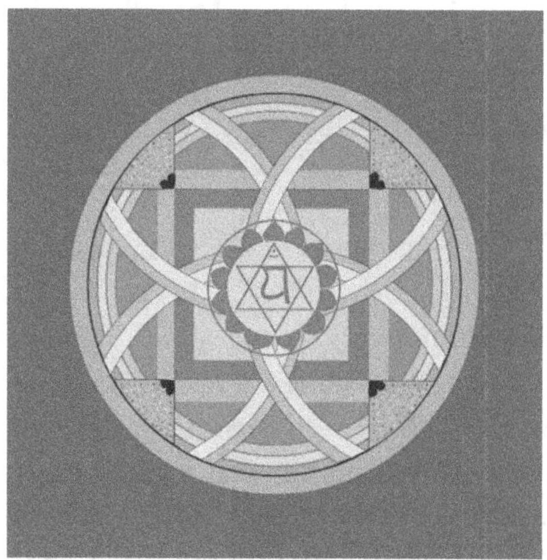

The Throat Chakra (Vishuddhi)

This is the fifth chakra in the sequence, located in front of the base of your neck. The hollow point in the center of your collar bones is the exact location of this chakra. This is the chakra that makes you immensely powerful. This chakra will empower you with the gift of expression and communication. People with powerful throat chakra can hold the masses with their gaze. They command undisputed authority and popularity. This is the chakra of the skilled and crafty people. It empowers you to master your craft with excellence. You get learning abilities like no one else in your genre. This is the chakra that can produce leaders of the masses. These are people with an amazing gift of words. Even your presence would speak volumes about your power in the room.

This is one of the most powerful chakras in the body. The power of this chakra resides in the fact that this chakra can also give you metaphysical powers. This may look like an exaggeration to a beginner, but it is an established fact that power in this chakra can increase your sense of perception. This means that you will be able to feel things that others can't. You will be able to feel not only tangible things in this world but also the intangible ones. Your perception of things increases energy levels. It means you will be able to feel the presence of different kinds of energies around you. It may also empower you to harness these energies for various chores. If you want to enhance your psychic abilities, then this is also the chakra you should be working on. If the third eye chakra is active in you, your psychic abilities will improve tremendously.

The third eye is the second chakra from the top, and it is highly focused on spiritual consciousness. This means the power in this chakra will help your understanding of spiritual matters.

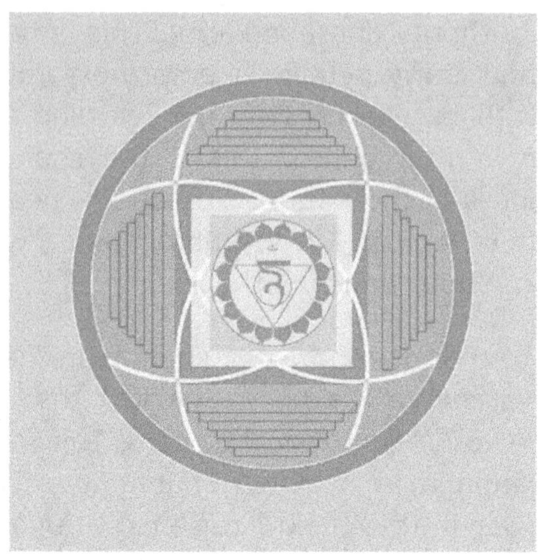

Third Eye Chakra (Ajna)

This is the sixth chakra and is called the third eye chakra. It is located in the middle of the forehead, between the eyebrows. This is a very spiritual chakra and is connected to the metaphysical world. It helps you connect to your higher self, and develop and nurture psychic abilities such as telepathy, astral travel, scrying, sensing events yet to happen, and connecting to past lives. The third eye is also an especially strong link between the spiritual and physical strength. A balanced third eye chakra can help improve your intuition and mental and spiritual clarity, strengthen your faith, make it easier for you to receive and accept spiritual guidance, and understand yourself on a much higher level. It can also encourage you to become more selfless, and increase your potential to develop psychic skills more easily and at a faster rate.

The third eye chakra is connected to the eyes, pituitary gland, endocrine system, and brain. Typical physical manifestations of an imbalanced third eye chakra are eye-related problems such as blurry vision or pain, sleeping disorders, headaches or migraines, and learning disabilities.

The third eye crystal is linked to the color indigo and the element of light. It is depicted by a two-petaled lotus.

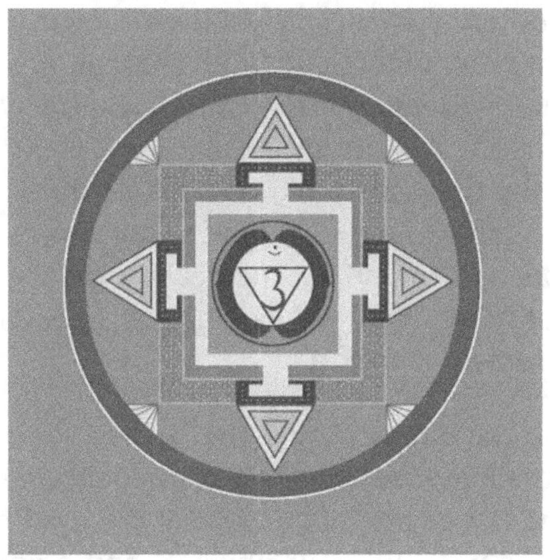

The Crown Chakra (Sahasrara)

This is the seventh chakra, and it is located at the top of your head. The physical location of this chakra is not inside your body but exactly on top of it. This is the chakra you should be working on if spiritual consciousness is your goal. If this chakra is powerful in your body, you will find this world to be very small for yourself. You will be full of energy and have the abilities to look beyond the visible things. This chakra gives you several abilities for you to feel more intellectually and spiritually realized. If this chakra becomes powerful, your physical aspirations diminish, and your spiritual hunger gets stronger. You will be the person who can ponder over the big questions of life and enlighten the world with pure knowledge.

These seven chakras hold the key to human consciousness. They regulate and influence our behavior. They have the ability to make us feel good, as well as pathetic. If your chakras are balanced and in harmony with each other, you may feel blessed even with limited means. However, if some of your chakras are blocked or out of sync, you may feel pathetic, even with all the material wealth at your disposal. They have everything they need, yet they feel a big void inside them. They keep looking for that one thing, which can make them feel complete but never find it. The reason for their failure is their misdirection. They are looking for a solution outside, while the problem is inside.

Ideally, the chakras should be active and balanced. However, the chakras function on a delicate balance of energy. This is heavily influenced by the kind of food you eat, your lifestyle, and your physical and emotional state as well. It is not very uncommon to have an imbalance in the chakras. Some chakras in the body can start functioning hyperactively. This happens when your inclination toward a particular thing grows very strongly. A chakra can start under-functioning when you start avoiding a particular thing or trait associated with that chakra. All such things keep happening inside the body, as energy is always in motion. However, if a chakra remains imbalanced, blocked, or hyperactive for very long, it can affect the functioning of your other chakras, too. Remember, all chakras are connected to each other. So, if one chakra is not working properly, it would affect the flow of energy in the body. The physical organs influenced by that chakra would also get affected.

Therefore, it is very important that you clearly understand the impact of chakras on your body and the influence they can have if there is an imbalance in the chakras. This will help you in preventing problems in life.

This book will help you in understanding chakras and the profound impact the chakras have on your character, personality, behavior, and functioning. You will get to know the ways in which imbalance in chakras can create havoc in your life and the techniques to balance the chakras.

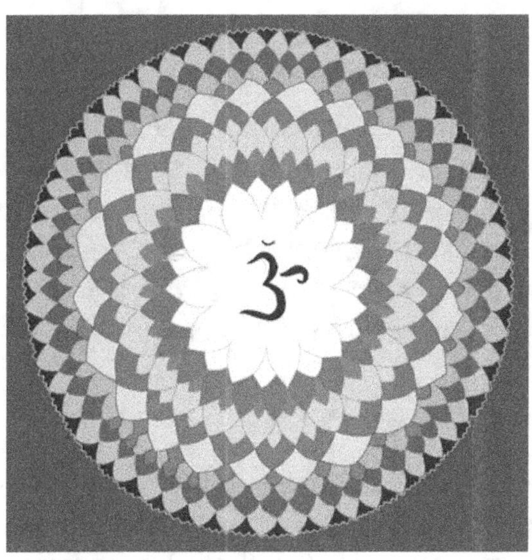

Chapter 17.
Chakra Meditation

Choosing a Meditation

Before deciding which meditation you want to practice, you'll first need to determine which chakras you'll focus your energy on, which chakra to start with, and in which order to address the other chakras. You'll also want to evaluate the timeframe you have to work with for the day and then set aside time in your schedule for meditation.

ONE CHAKRA OR MANY?

The order won't negatively affect any of your other chakras. However, a good general rule is to work on the chakra with the most issues first. I recommend that you listen to your intuition to determine which chakra is giving you the most trouble.

Some chakra experts prefer to work from the center out, because the central chakras—heart and solar plexus— tend to become "stuck" due to their locations. Another option is to start with the root space and then move up to the crown. Opening these end chakras usually will bring about a big shift, so your energy can flow and balance can naturally return.

I prefer to work on the heart chakra first because this chakra is the ultimate connection to your infinite being. I usually find that once the heart chakra is cleared, energy issues within other chakras are easier to resolve. For example, say I am experiencing emotional pain from a breakup, and because I have not dealt with those feelings, I am also experiencing anxiety and back pain. My solar plexus is being affected as well as my heart space. I would first want to focus on heart-based healing and then on my solar plexus to address my physical symptoms.

TIME AS A FACTOR

The meditations in this book fit into 5-, 15-, or 30-minute time-frames to make finding a meditation that will suit your schedule easy. The five-minute meditations are a nice way to dip your toes in the water before you get into the deep end. They are also perfect for energetic maintenance. The longer meditations will help you unlock your creativity and examine personal connections in deep and profound ways. They will yield great insights, clarity, and focus and make your practice more meaningful.

To really clear a chakra on your own, without Reiki or the use of other energy modalities, you'll want to sit with that specific chakra for a minimum of 30 to 45 minutes. You'll have the option to extend all of the meditations in this book with additional breathing and visualization exercises. Time is of the essence, so choose your meditation wisely and commit to it for the minimum suggested length to receive the full benefits.

WHAT'S YOUR INTENTION?

Setting an intention before you begin meditating is the perfect way to formalize what you want to achieve. An intention also improves your odds of successfully making your wish a reality. For example, you may want to achieve balance. Maybe you want a more harmonious relationship with yourself or another person. Perhaps you have an urgent health issue. Maybe you're tackling a bigger issue, such as what you want most out of your life.

Whatever your need, just remember that a restorative or preventative long-term practice will look and feel different than a practice that directly addresses an immediate need, such as a health crisis. Be sure to check in with yourself before you start each meditation in order to determine your goals. If your intention shifts once you get started, simply adjust. Being open and flexible is how all seasoned meditators achieve the greatest results.

The Elements of Guided Meditation

There are many ways to explore your meditation practice, including mantras, visualizations, breath work, and reflections. You may find it beneficial to begin by practicing a few meditations with a friend. You may also find it beneficial to record yourself reading the meditation instructions so you can play them back whenever you need a reminder.

If you feel called to make one of the mantras the focus of your meditation, you could potentially do a full sit with that mantra and challenge yourself with a timer. You don't have to pair any meditation elements in order for a meditation to be coherent and successful. Once you learn the foundational elements of meditation, you can put them together however you see fit. The beauty of this practice is that it is yours.

MANTRAS AND MUDRA

In Sanskrit, the word mantra can be broken into two parts: man, which means "mind," and tra, which means "vehicle." Therefore, a mantra is essentially a vehicle of the mind, a type of spiritual formula used to quickly take you into a deep state of meditation.

Mantras help you alter your state of consciousness. Chanting a powerful word or phrase, every syllable of which is specifically designed to affect subconscious impulses and habits, helps you transcend thought and heighten your awareness.

Mudras are hand postures or gestures that are practiced with your fingers, and their origins are rooted in Hinduism and Buddhism. Because your hand is mapped to your brain, mudras target the reflex points important for unlocking certain biological signals such as relaxation, metabolic rate, or circulation. Adding mudras to your meditations is not necessary but can complement and enhance your practice.

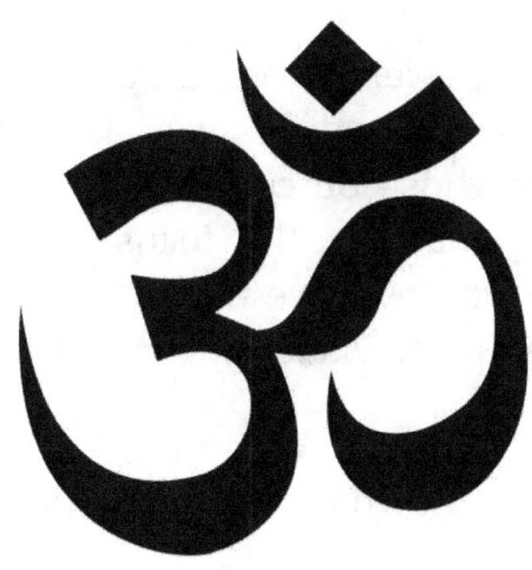

The symbol of Oṃ, the most sacred Hindu mantra

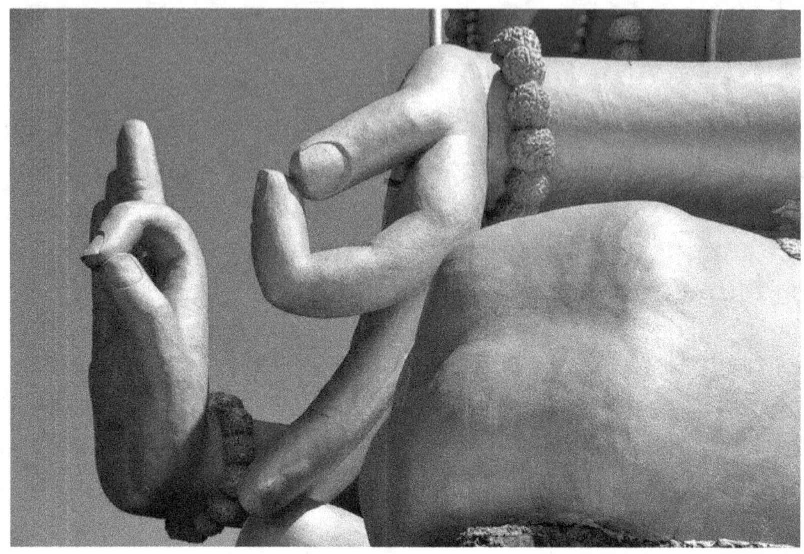

The hands form the Dhyanamudra

VISUALIZATION

Many meditations in this book include some type of visualization. Some visualizations involve specific colors or ask you to use your imagination to enhance your experience. But the emphasis should always be on the feeling that the visualization evokes.

Visualization is a powerful meditation tool that's used to influence the physical body as well as desired outcomes, particularly when those outcomes involve health. Deepak Chopra teaches whatever the focus of our attention, it grows stronger; whatever we withdraw our attention from diminishes. Therefore, visualizing wellness creates more of it.

Visualizations are known to manifest specific results with

startling accuracy. Creating a mental image of desired feelings and situations helps you elicit them. Use this practice to live in ways that support your desired goals.

Everything is created twice. First in the mind, and then in reality.

—ROBIN S. SHARMA

MEDITATION

For each chakra, I'll guide you through meditations that are 5, 15, and 30 minutes in length and that instruct you to link your breath with color and other visualizations. The bulk of the meditations focus on the areas, systems, and organs of the body that each chakra governs. By regularly practicing these meditations, you'll get to know each chakra intimately, and you'll create your desired healing effect.

I'll be asking a lot of you in these meditations, especially if you're practicing chakra healing for the first time. But don't worry—I'll provide tips. I'll also explain how to expand the shorter meditations.

CLOSING REFLECTION

Engaging in reflection will help you get comfortable with building your awareness so you can be more in tune with your body and your mind.

After your meditation has concluded, spend about five minutes putting ideas or thoughts that you need to process onto paper. You could also sit with the newly created space of awareness that comes up during meditation. Either way is fine.

Although you won't be cued to spend time in reflection after every meditation, it's a good idea to set two timers: one for the length of the meditation and one for five minutes longer, to give yourself a little buffer before coming back to the real world.

Monkey Mind

The mind can be a land mine of distractions and activity. Your thoughts can race around—much like monkeys swinging from tree to tree. The trees in this case are your emotions and thoughts that are attempting to gain your attention. Originally a Buddhist term meaning "unsettled," "restless," or "indecisive," monkey mind can refer to any mind chatter.

Meditation is not about stopping the chatter—rather, it's about making a choice. Each time you drop into meditation, you have a choice: Allow distractions to pull you out of your space or show up for yourself and go deeper into that space. Instead of jumping from branch to branch, giving anything and everything your attention, make the choice to be present and quiet the chaos.

That choice doesn't mean that you should ignore the chatter. In fact, acknowledging your thoughts can neutralize them, particularly when they include self-doubt.

Giving your mind a task is a good way to transcend thought patterns and processes. One simple technique is to focus on your breath moving in and out of your body. If you become overwhelmed by monkey mind, try incorporating a mantra into your meditation.

Over time, you'll become better at being in the moment.

With practice, your thoughts will become less disruptive. Consistency is key here. It's all about training your monkey mind so you can swing gracefully through the trees with patience, compassion, and control.

Before You Begin

Before jumping into your healing practice, there are a few steps that need to be covered. Some of these may seem a bit obvious, but I wouldn't be doing my due diligence as a healer if I didn't include them.

Clearing some time for your meditation is imperative to ensure that your practice is successful. Try setting a daily reminder on your phone to help you establish a meditation habit. Make sure you are comfortable. Eliminate distractions and plan time for reflection before your meditation starts. I'll go over these steps in more detail below.

Do a general check-in with yourself to connect with your current emotions. Make note of any issues so you can develop a loving attitude of self-acceptance each time you practice meditation. And don't worry about whether you're doing it wrong, because there is no wrong way to meditate—I promise!

WHAT YOU'LL NEED

Although meditation doesn't cost money, it does take commitment. The amount of time and effort you put into your practice determines its success.

Outside distractions are all part of the meditation. However, minimize interruptions as much as possible. Make sure you won't be disrupted by any electronics during your sit time. Silence your phone before you begin.

You'll want to keep this book nearby so you can take quick peeks if you get lost during a sit, especially when you're first starting your meditation practice. If you keep a meditation journal, have it easily accessible post-sit.

REFLECTION

It's natural for feelings to come up during meditation. You may need time post-sit to process and integrate these feelings. Creating space for reflection after each meditation is a good practice. I won't give reflection reminders at the end of each meditation, but you'll want to note how you feel.

If some action items have made themselves apparent during your meditation, you can create a to-do list. Drawing or sketching a solution in a journal is another option. A meditation journal can help you succinctly acknowledge whatever came up for you. Plus, it's a great tool for tracking your progress.

On the other hand, it's okay if you feel that not much transpired. It may take a few days or weeks to fully integrate what actually went on behind the scenes during a sit. The solution may be a longer sit.

Reconciling Emotions

When you finish a meditation, you may experience unsettling emotions. When you tap into your subconscious mind, energy begins to move and clear, and you may come away with feelings of frustration, sadness, pain, or anger. Consider meditation an opportunity to integrate and release these feelings.

Although most of us do not like to admit it, pain and discomfort are vital aspects of the human experience. Pain is a response to something occurring in your reality, whereas suffering is the choice to prolong that pain. Both are unpleasant experiences, but they offer a tremendous opportunity for growth, and they remind us of the balance we need to reach our highest potential.

To escape suffering, remember that you have the power to view things from a different perspective. Consistent meditation can help you make that shift. We may not understand why something is happening, but we can do our best to trust, surrender, and accept our emotions—even if they come in the form of pain and suffering.

Taking notes and acknowledging how you feel will help make sense of your healing journey. Consistent reflection will help you build trust in yourself so you'll feel confident listening to your body and mind when they speak—even if they whisper.

Getting Comfortable

You will want to dress in comfortable clothing. Nothing is worse than being pulled away from your meditation by an itchy sweater or too-tight jeans. If you are meditating before work or during lunch, make adjustments that will help you relax, like removing your belt or settling into a cozy chair.

It's not necessary to use a professional meditation cushion, but you will want some back support for comfort. Worrying about discomfort draws attention away from your awareness, so eliminating that issue beforehand will only help facilitate your journey.

When you sit, whether on the floor or in a chair, a straight spine is ideal. If seated on the floor, your legs can be in the lotus position, folded, or straight out in front of you. If you are seated in a chair, your feet should be flat on the floor. I do not recommend crossing your legs or arms because it impedes the flow of energy through your body. If you want to lie down for the meditation, make sure you do so at a time of day when you're likely to remain alert.

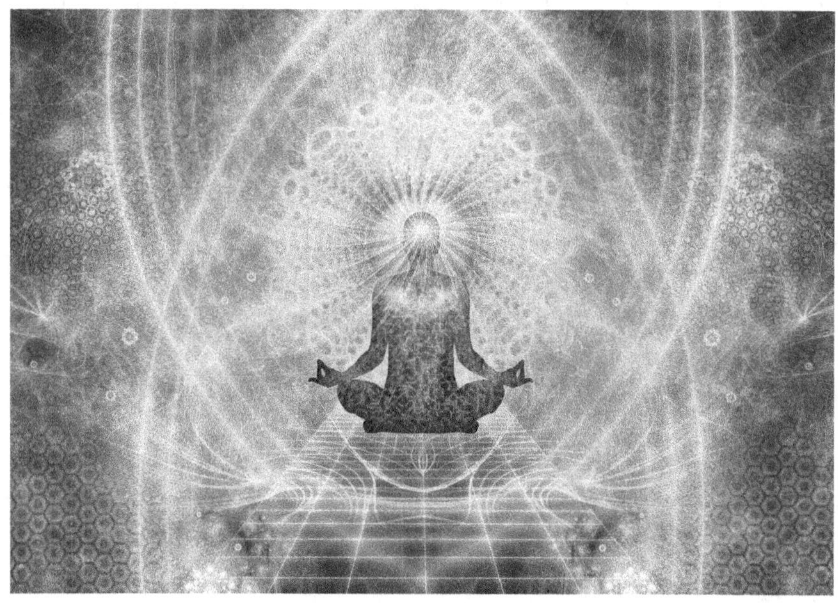

Chapter 18.
Healing Your Chakras

Using the methods of chakra healing, you can treat numerous physical ailments that weren't caused by medical problems or injuries. Pain and diseases that root in mental causes, instead of medical, are called psychosomatic. They are called this because they signal mental distress. They are a sign that your body is overrun by stress hormones and fear hormones. However, it's not enough for you to acknowledge that some of your ailments come from your mind. To understand which particular aspects of your emotional life are struck with blockage and denial and to learn how to release them, you can look into each individual symptom and tie it to the corresponding mental problems.

With this information, you'll understand your body better, and you'll know which of your symptoms result from emotional and spiritual problems.

Headache

If you're suffering from chronic headaches without obvious medical causes, it could be due to the imbalance in your third eye chakra and the crown chakra.

Chronic headaches, followed by sinus pressure, and the pressure in the back part of your head and your eyes, that spread across your forehead, are the most typical sign of the disharmony in the third eye chakra.

These pains are a signal that you are mainly focusing on the intellectual and neglecting the spiritual aspects of your existence. You may be afraid of your spiritual aspects. Because of this, you are ignoring your intuitive hints and abandoning the wisdom of your third eye.

Many times, your instincts tell you to do things that seem to go against logic. You feel these signals, but you are afraid that acting on them would be risky. For example, if you unconsciously feel like you should quit your job, but there is no new job in sight, you might be ignoring this instinct.

Subconsciously, your third eye knows the things that are beyond your conscious knowledge. It might be signaling to you that the better opportunity is coming your way. Or, you may be in the presence of a person you unconsciously know has a negative effect on you. But, you are ignoring the intuitive signals to stay away from that person.

On the other hand, a headache at the top center of your head is often a sign of the imbalance in the crown chakra. This type of headache suggests difficulty trusting the intuitive signs regarding your life path.

You may fear that acting and living in accordance with the Divine signals will lead to something risky or irresponsible. This results from having difficulties in seeing a larger picture and cultivating your faith in yourself and in the Divine.

Fatigue

Fatigue is detrimental to your energy focus and concentration which all results in low motivation. If you are someone who usually overwork themselves into exhaustion, you are overloading your solar plexus chakra and your power center is being overstimulated.

If you're suffering from fatigue, it is most likely due to the imbalance in the crown chakra and the solar plexus chakra. The ongoing exhaustion that only increases and doesn't go away after rest, with a constant feeling of weariness and low energy, signals chakra imbalance.

This can happen if you are associating achievement and self-esteem with the quality of your performance. If you feel like failing to deliver quality performance makes you unworthy, it can have a negative effect on your solar plexus chakra. This is often followed by low self-esteem, depression, and loss of faith in the Divine.

Stomach disorders

Pain and uncomfortable symptoms in your stomach come from the imbalance of the solar plexus chakra. Diseases related to stomach include diarrhea, constipation, intestinal problems, ulcers, acid reflux, and many others. If you are certain that you haven't eaten any foods that might have upset your stomach, or that there haven't been any physical injuries that might have caused these symptoms, you can inspect your solar plexus chakra to see if it's out of balance.

Pain in your stomach can often result from the feeling of powerlessness, a sense of overwhelm, a perception that you are losing control of your life, feeling intimidated or having low self-respect. If you went through significant changes in your life, like a divorce, problematic relationships with other people, or a loss of a job, these experiences could have produced a lot of anger, resentment, guilt, and other toxic emotions.

If your self-esteem is compromised, you will have a very toxic combination of negative feelings towards other people and yourself. The key to resolving this is to forgive both yourself and others, as well as admitting that there is no reason to place blame on anyone.

To overcome stomach pains related to the solar plexus chakra, you can apply the solar plexus meditation or use essential oils to treat your stomach area with more kindness and compassion.

Psychosomatic digestive problems arise from your problems with processing stress. They are a sign that you are ignoring to resolve problems in your daily life. When you're not processing daily stresses, they become suppressed. You are resorting to emotional avoidance.

As a result of this, you are closing your solar plexus chakra because you don't want to deal with problems.

This is dangerous because your solar plexus is the center of your personal power. When you avoid confronting problems, you are shutting yourself out from using your personal power to solve them. As a result of this, you feel frightened, powerless, and your self-esteem is low. The only solution for this is addressing the things that are bothering you.

Detachment

When you feel disconnected and detached from yourself and the world around you that means that you've closed your heart chakra. In this state, you abandon your passions and you give up everything that makes you happy and fulfilled.

The first sign of the imbalance of the heart chakra is the lack of connection with others. You may feel the need to be alone, which can turn into isolation. When you feel the need to isolate from others, it means that you are shutting yourself out.

You want to feel happy and joyful, but it seems like you are no longer able to. You are out of touch with everything that makes you happy. This can lead to depression.

You may even be disconnected from your physical body and unable to feel the physical sensations before they become overwhelming. For example, you don't notice symptoms of illnesses before they become too intense. You start living on autopilot, disengaging from your true self.

Detachment is best treated with mindfulness. Start looking into everything that makes you happy. Focus on gratefulness and put more effort into spending time with your friends and family. First, you need to establish a good connection with yourself, which can be done through meditation and other self-care practices.

Depression

While physical trauma can induce depression, it is mainly a mental state in which a person's negative beliefs prevail over the positive perceptions of oneself and life. What gives people a sense of purpose, meaning, and a feeling that they belong in the world is faith in God. Having faith in God is essential because none of us are truly in control over anything, including our own lives and our own bodies.

What keeps us going is the faith that there is general positivity in the world and that things will work out for us. We rely on this faith even when outside manifestation speaks otherwise.

Due to traumatic events, a problematic childhood, or a combination of multiple factors, negative beliefs can prevail over positive thoughts. When you have experiences like these, your heart chakra and your crown chakra will fall out of balance.

Your heart chakra is in charge of being open to love. It is in charge of feeling worthy of love and wanting to love others selflessly and unconditionally. Related to that is the crown chakra, which embodies your relationship with the Divine. That relationship is primarily a relationship of love. It requires faith.

When you fall into depression, you essentially lose faith in love. Not only in love, you lose faith in "good," which resonates with losing faith in God. This is an unconscious process that might not manifest in conscious thoughts due to blockage. You don't want to admit that you've lost your faith and you block out these feelings.

As a result, you feel hopeless and undeserving of anything good. In this state, both your crown and heart chakra will close or constrict. You will experience continuous sadness, feeling hopeless, and empty. You will have trouble finding pleasure and feel like your life is not worth living.

This condition also affects your appetite and sleep, which puts you in an even worse situation. Your energy comes from the foods you consume, and when you're neglecting your diet, you are also depriving yourself of the source of your life energy. You become energetically depleted.

The crown chakra, when out of balance, produces a feeling of loneliness. In extreme situations, this can lead to suicidal thoughts, and eventually suicide.

When you are feeling depressed, focus on working on balancing your heart chakra first. Your heart chakra helps you open up to love. It helps you open up to the sense of safety. It also helps you accept the idea that you are worthy of unconditional love and that there's nothing that you have to do to deserve it.

Your crown chakra, which should only be treated when the root chakra is in good shape, is now in need of love. To work on your crown chakra, devote to religious, mindful, or spiritual practices. You should work on your relationship with the Divine, in whichever ways you practice spiritual beliefs.

Make sure to address any unconscious anger towards God. Most people find it hard to grasp that while God is a cosmic force that teaches you about right and wrong, He is also endlessly forgiving. When people feel guilty, they also feel like God thinks they are guilty, and God is judging them. This is never true. The Divine force is the force of unconditional forgiveness.

If you feel angry with God, you actually feel angry at yourself. You assume that God is angry at you because you didn't act according to his/her/its teachings.

In this case, you should contemplate on God's imminent and unconditional love for every person. You can do this by reading scriptures or talking to a religious teacher who will explain how the Divine looks at people, and why it always forgives.

Grief

Loss can cause constriction and the closing of the heart chakra.

Grief is a feeling that results from losing something that is precious to us. With relationships, jobs, and material goods, it's easier to cope with grief because there is a lesser significance to the loss. However, some losses, like the death of loved ones and children are very hard to cope with. There's no replacement for what we're missing, and relief seems impossible to find.

Loss can very easily block your heart chakra, causing you to grief for a long time. This causes the feeling of loneliness, hopelessness, and the cultivation of bitterness.

Grief is commonly followed by isolation. In some cases, isolation is a good idea for you to rejuvenate and pick yourself up. However, if isolation results from the unwillingness to reconnect with the world, it can become harmful.

Your heart chakra connects you to the sense of self-love and love for others. Grief can cause you to lose faith in love, and even choose to detach from it, to avoid feeling pain. The cure for grief is reconnecting with your own inner feeling of self-love, love for others, and the outside world. If you feel like grief has become toxic for you, there are many healthy ways for you to reconnect.

You can start by practicing self-love and self-care and then move to connect with people, plants, and animals. If a heartbreak makes it hard for you to reconnect with your loved ones, you can start by connecting with plants and animals. Gradually, this connection will help you open up to connecting with people.

Guilt

An overwhelming feeling of guilt may constrict your solar plexus and the sacral plexus chakra. When you feel profoundly guilty of having done something wrong, whether or not this perception is true, you detach yourself from feeling pleasure. You deny yourself pleasure because you feel undeserving of it.

This can cause you to repress your sexuality, emotions, and overall detach from doing things that make you happy. Guilt results in the loss of will to express yourself in healthy ways.

To heal guilt, practice meditations for solar and sacral plexus chakras, and also work on healthy self-expression. Healing from guilt means being able to assume the responsibility for your actions but releasing the feeling of inadequacy.

No one benefits from you feeling guilty. The guilt itself

doesn't repair any harm that you may have done. You can work towards amending whatever harm you have done if there's room for it. If not, you can only work to learn from your mistakes. However, making a mistake doesn't mean that you no longer deserve to be happy.

Anxiety

Anxiety affects all chakras depending on the type of strain you're exposed to. Everyday life often entails a moderate amount of anxiety. However, long-term anxiety followed by constant stress can have a negative impact on your health. You will become more vulnerable to triggers. Within minutes of a triggering situation, you can find yourself in a state of panic.

Most often, anxiety affects your crown and heart chakra. This happens when you start to feel like God doesn't have your back. The third eye chakra causes anxiety due to fear of the unknown, and distrust of your intuition.

This can severely impact your quality of life. When your throat chakra is out of harmony, you will be anxious about expressing your opinions and holding your truth. As a result, everything you have to say and the things that burdens you will be repressed.

Holding on to past hurts can block your heart chakra and cause anxiousness because you feel disconnected from your own feelings. Intimidation and overwhelming fear, be it in the area of work, finance, or relationships, with the added pressure to perform perfectly, causes your solar plexus chakra to fall out of balance.

With sacral plexus chakra, anxiety results from feeling guilty and ashamed to confess your needs and insecurities. Over time, these built-up tensions can have a profoundly debilitating impact on your life. Anxiety also touches your root chakra in the form of feeling insecure and unsafe.

To heal anxiety using chakra healing, you should examine your insecurities in all aspects of your inner being, starting from the bottom to the top.

Screen all of your chakras and determine which areas are a source of negative energy. Then, start by practicing grounding to insure yourself that the Earth is supporting you. Proceed to heal your chakras using meditation, crystals, and essential oils. Focus on releasing your fears in regard to all issues that are relevant to the chakras.

Anger

Anger mostly affects your root chakra, but it also touches on the other energy centers as well. Anger, in its core, is a healthy feeling that drives you to stand up for yourself, establish boundaries, act, and initiate change.

However, anger can also become a tool for you to repress sadness. When this happens, you are using anger to defend yourself from the inner feeling of sadness and hopelessness. Fear can also be the root of anger and your using anger away to the fence yourself being afraid. While anger resonates deeply with the root chakra, it affects all other chakras. If you are angry at God for the suffering of bad faith, this touches on your crown chakra.

Your third eye also becomes affected because due to this, you lose faith in your own intuition. You're out of touch with an inner sense of emotional intelligence. You will become unable to trust yourself, and as a result, you no longer trust the world and the Divine. You also start to distrust your community and your loved ones. The key to healing anger is to inspect the underlying feelings.

For example, if you are angry for not standing up for yourself, the solution might be in balancing your solar plexus chakra. However, if you feel anger, to defend yourself from fear and sadness, the solutions are to treat your heart chakra and your sacral chakra. These chakras open you up to forgiveness and love.

If your anger roots in feeling burdened, then it's possible that you are holding in some truths that need to be said. These truths can relate to many areas of your life, from unpleasant things that you need to admit to yourself to deeply hidden truths you want to reveal to the world. If guilt and shame stop you from doing this, you need to learn how to overcome them. Only when you start going through life fully authentic to your inner truth will you be able to relieve the anger and live in peace.

Chapter 19.
The Third Eye And
Your Psychic Awakening

The third eye is the main ascension space when you are preparing to reach enlightenment. You cannot begin to even wonder what it means to be enlightened if your third eye is blocked, congested, or stagnant. The third eye is the seat of perception, intuition, and "clear knowing," and it is how we are wonderfully able to connect to our dreams and visions in a more profound way.

You can live your whole life without ever knowing the quality of what it feels like to be connected to this part of yourself, and many people describe it as feeling high without having any drugs or alcohol. It can be the way that you ask yourself to pursue a higher mind so that you can live a fuller life, which sometimes means letting go of the status quo and not trying so hard to "fit in."

Answering the call of the third eye isn't as hard as people might suggest, and when you are open to it and have created awareness about it, you can begin to use simple tools to help yourself realize the power of the third eye in your overall chakra healing experience.

Mental Relaxation Tools to Awaken Higher Consciousness

Your mind is a machine, constantly computing and deciding, deciphering and learning, and even feeling skeptical or judgmental. Your third eye doesn't have time for all of that and will have a harder time being open if you are closed off to it with your mental thoughts. The third eye is energy, and it is the beginning of your worlds becoming one, between the physical and the spiritual.

The mental attitudes and beliefs that people adopt in early life, or adapt to within their culture or community, can be very limiting to the third eye and so as you prepare to work with opening this energy, it is important to find ways to relax your mind in order to awaken higher consciousness.

Mindfulness is a form of meditation that can be performed in any situation. It is an act of being totally conscious of everything that you are experiencing at the moment without letting your mind wander too far into the past or the future. It keeps your mind free of anxious or worrisome thoughts because you are working only to engage with the experience you are having right now.

Mindfulness can take some practice, and it is incredibly simple to learn. All you have to do is follow these simple guidelines:

- Focus and concentrate on what you are working with right now.

- Don't get caught up in making assumptions or having too many opinions about the experience. Try to just enjoy a quiet mind while you take in the situation or surroundings.

- Find the openings you see in your intuition and let them guide you forward. Trust your instinct.

- When your mind starts to churn too much, or worry what others might be doing, thinking and feeling, return yourself to what you are doing and give it added focus.

- Breathe, inhales and exhales, steadily and calmly.

- Give yourself over to going with the flow and don't try to control the situation or the outcomes.

- Visualize your inner world as it is making contact with your outer world and see how the two can be together. Practice seeing more than what your eyes can see naturally.

These simple guidelines are just some of the basics of practicing mindfulness. When you are working to incorporate a higher consciousness level of thinking and processing information, you have to be able to let go of control and just bear witness to reality. It will show you what you need to know, rather than imposing an opinion, belief, or attitude upon it.

This is the platform for thinking from a higher state of being, and it will naturally occur that your third eye will expand and become more alive to your overall thought process naturally as a result of this attitude or process.

The Art of Creative Visualization

To be able to see with your eyes closed is the gift of the third eye. It is not something reserved only for the enlightened. It is possible for any person, no matter what level of awakening they are involved with at the moment. All it takes is a little effort and a few minutes of your time to practice this useful skill.

Creative visualization feels a lot like what it is like to dream. When you go to sleep at night, and you can recall your dreams, there are usually moving pictures, images, sensations, and even thoughts or words. When you are creatively visualizing something out of the dream state, you are activating your higher mind and deeper consciousness.

There are plenty of people who already know how to do this and have always known how to close their eyes and imagine a far off and fantastical landscape full of whatever comes to mind. With a little practice, it can become even more detailed and elaborate, and you will find a greater opening with your capabilities with your psychic visions and ability to see beyond what is visible to the naked eye.

It is this skill that will help you see your chakras more clearly and be more open to understanding the visions that come up or resurface from past experiences so that you know what you need to let go of clearly. The path of awakening the third eye can be advanced when you practice this technique. Here are the simple guidelines to follow when you are practicing creative visualization:

- Be open to anything that might surface without judgment or criticism.

- Let go of thought patterns and cycles that you might easily get stuck in (ex: "I can't," "that isn't real/possible," "It doesn't even make any sense," etc.).

- Teach yourself your own methods and avoid looking online or in books for a guide to help you connect with your third eye. The point is that you are connecting to your own unique intuition and identity.

- Visualize things simple at first and then more elaborately as you get better at seeing the minute details.

- Practice traveling to other "inner landscapes" and worlds to help show yourself the metaphorical and symbolic path that you need to travel.

- Design your worlds to be places that you can return to over and over again to help yourself along your healing path.

- Use your thoughts and feelings to direct the course of your creative visualization. It will help you to better identify what chakras will need the most healing, balance, or strengthening.

These simple guidelines are just to give you a platform to begin your own creative work. The journey of awakening the third eye is unique to the individual and will be different for everyone. It is important not to get too boxed into other people's views or perspectives about the "right" or "wrong" way to open your third eye (or any other chakras, for that matter).

Creative visualization is a portal to help you understand your own inner truth as well as to finding your path to universal consciousness and enlightenment.

Power of Psychic Awareness Through the Third Eye

There are no limits to what the human mind is capable of. We are only limited by our beliefs and ideas about what it all is supposed to be or look like. Awakening, the third eye asks you to let go of all of your preconceived notions of reality and to step into a new way of seeing all life on the planet.

The power of psychic awareness will make it challenging for you to know anything the way that you knew it before. It causes a great shift in your ability to "see" and "know" the truth about all areas of your life, which will, in turn, cause a lot of change, even when it is uncomfortable. You may not know it yet, but when you begin to ascend into your psychic knowledge, you will look at your world with a new set of eyes, and it will suddenly feel like everything you are doing in your life right now is "off" and needs to change or be resolved.

This great transformation happens very quickly, and many people will even avoid the cost of letting it unfold naturally out of fear of such a big life change or shift in consciousness and identity. There are certainly ways that you can help this experience unfold in a healthier and more comfortable way and here are just a few tips to help you understand that process:

- Give up anything that no longer makes you feel like yourself.

- Look for ways to explore your psychic awareness by listening to your inner codes and messages that come up. It is your intuition and inner knowing speaking to you. Keep a journal or a record of these psychic thoughts.

- Bring yourself into a state of trance or meditation on a daily or regular basis to help you expand your consciousness more effectively.

- Take a moment to listen to your gut reactions and instincts before you make a choice or speak any words to someone or yourself.

- Denial is not a helpful tool, and so if you ask these questions and receive a response, do not deny it, no matter how far-fetched it may seem.

- Collaborate with other methods of psychic practice, such as divination, scrying, tarot card reading, crystal empowerment of the third eye, etc.

- Release any beliefs that suggest that being psychic isn't real or true.

The moment you begin to embrace your ability to just "know" you are giving yourself the opening to awakening your psychic abilities more than ever before. What are those psychic abilities? They manifest differently for everyone, but here is a list of some possibilities:

- Prophetic dreams and prophecies

- The ability to see what is about to happen as it is about to happen

- Welcoming the presence of spirit guides and other "ethereal helpers."

- Clairvoyance and clairsentience

- Being able to predict possible outcomes in a detailed way

- Journeying in mind to other dimensions of reality, or astral travel

- Being able to speak to energies on the "other side."

- Reading auras and being able to see the light and coloration of the auras

- Being able to read another person's energy and interpret what they are not saying out loud

- Telepathy

- And more!

Psychic awareness takes a lot of personal growth, stamina, and ability to see beyond the third dimension of reality. It can take you years to uncover the depths of your psychic powers and path, and if you put in the work to truly know yourself in this way, then you can advance your soulful awakening even faster than if you just did a few things here and a couple of things there.

Understanding Enlightenment

Enlightenment simply means that you are awakening to your whole light source and power as a person. It is a connection to the universally divine energies inherent in all things and all nature. You don't have to be a yoga guru or someone who lives and breathes the philosophies of Eastern religions in order to know enlightenment. It is a different path for every person with different ways of traveling throughout life.

There are a lot of ways that people will feel confused about what enlightenment is because they are looking for perfection. It is not a state of perfection that equals enlightenment, but rather a state of truth within your own being. If you are resistant to your own truth, then you are not likely to become fully enlightened, and in order to get to that connection with yourself, you have to let go of what you think and believe that the world wants you to be. You can live your whole life exhausting your true purpose by trying to fit in the way other people do or try to.

Enlightenment is a growth experience, and it will never fit into a list of rules or a checklist. It is an ongoing process that delivers you to your highest and purest form of consciousness and even that required continuous fine-tuning and exploration. There really is no endpoint to the journey of self-discovery, and it will only limit you if you think, feel or believe that if only you could just make it that point, everything will be great forever.

It simply won't work that way, and having an awakened mind means that you are already in awareness of that simple truth and reality. Your third eye and your psychic ascension is the path that opens you to becoming enlightened and working forward toward living your life by your inner light and source energy. And that is really what healing the chakras and awakening is all about in the first place.

Chapter 20.
The Ways To Protect Yourself During Third Eye Activation

The third eye activation is a powerful process. It makes you more receptive. You will attract energies around you. However, you cannot have real control over the kind of energies with which you may come in contact. You simply become the receiver of energies. This can pose a problem.

The positive energies will bring peace and tranquility. They will make you strong and blissful. However, negative energies can have a stronger but negative impact. To this end, it is important that you protect yourself. You must become aware of the energies around you. You must choose the place of practice carefully. You should also work to seal your aura for getting better protection against negative energies.

Neglecting these important aspects can have serious consequences on your physical, mental, as well as spiritual health. Enabling psychic protection against negative energies is the best way to avoid these issues.

The places of meditation, the lifestyle you follow, and even the kind of clothes you wear have important roles to play in your protection. Proper attention to all these aspects will help you in ensuring proper protection. We will now discuss the main things that you need to take into consideration.

The Place

The place of meditation has a very important role to play in ensuring your protection. We are surrounded by all kinds of energies. There are positive energies that help us in our endeavors. There are negative energies that push us down or corner us. The whole concept of things and places being lucky or unlucky isn't just a misconception. When positive energies in a place are dominant, that place becomes lucky. It helps you in becoming successful. You become more energetic and alive. Your entrepreneurial skills get sharp. Your risk-taking abilities become stronger. Your ability to judge people, things, and circumstances gets better. You feel rejuvenated and healthy. However, if the place is dominated by negative energies, things are exactly the opposite.

Therefore, ignoring the significance of the place is not a very prudent thing. We are not the first to roam on this earth. Several people have walked, lived, and died in the same place where we live at present. A part of their energy is left behind. Accumulation of such energies has a profound effect on the nature of that place.

This earth is the place from which we all have originated. It is also a very powerful source of energy. It is full of energies that are so powerful that your body can never react to them positively. Such energies keep leaking from the fault lines. If you are at a place which is contaminated by such energies, then they will have a negative impact on you. Fear, health, and psychological problems are only some type of issues that can be faced.

In the past, people gave great significance to the earth's energies. They had the luxury to move things around. Space was ample. They could shift even a home if it rested on such fault lines. Modern lifestyle doesn't permit you this luxury. Living spaces have become smaller. Homes have become so expensive that shifting them in search of a feasible option isn't an option anymore. However, there are other remedies like Feng Shui, Vastu Shashtra, dowsing, house healing, and other such practices that can help you in cultivating positive energies. You will be able to identify the places in your home filled with negative energies. Such places can be easily avoided, and you can do constructive practices elsewhere. Like fields of negative energies, homes also have energy wells. These are the areas of positive energy. You can identify these areas and utilize them to your advantage.

Earth ray lines have been known to be a reason for several health issues. Our ancestor's associated cot deaths with such ray lines. People sleeping on these ray lines are known to be prone to joint problems, heart conditions, migraine headaches, and other such ailments. Frequent and unexplained bed-wetting is also attributed to these ray lines. If you are constantly having bad dreams while sleeping in the same place, then changing the direction or position of your bed can help. Insomnia or difficulty in sleeping can be due to this problem.

Such energies also impact your meditation and its results. While you are in a meditative state, your aura expands, and it starts communicating with the energies around it. Excessive influence of negative energies can lead to fear and visualization of negative imagery. It can leave you in a fearful state and make longer meditations difficult. That's why it is important to find a place that is more conducive.

Once you start meditation, your sense of perception will become sharper. You will be able to feel such energies strongly. If you feel that meditating at any particular place is getting difficult, you must change the place. You can also take the help of professional dowsers, house healers, or Feng Shui to balance the energies.

Work on Yourself

A healthy body and a balanced mind are the best defense

Attacking the weak is the best strategy and we all know this. Negativity will engulf the weak of mind and body first. So, you must always focus on having a healthy body and a balanced mind. If you remain healthy and sane, negative forces will not be able to influence you easily. You must adopt a healthy lifestyle to remain protected.

A balanced lifestyle and mindset are the first requisite for any such practice. If you are stepping into your practice with a negative outlook, the results won't be very promising. Your journey would remain bumpy, and you would face several impediments on the way.

A healthy body is a strong foundation for success. You will be able to face your fears with strength and overpower the roadblocks easily. The protection techniques will work in any condition, but a healthy lifestyle will help you in many ways.

Third eye activation is a spiritual journey, but it has to be carried out through your physical body; and therefore, you can never ignore the importance of your physicality. You must take steps to ensure that you remain healthy and focused. Following a healthy lifestyle will take you a long way in this process.

Sleep and rest are important

An exhausted body is weak and prone to the influence of negative energies. If you are taxing yourself too much or not getting enough sleep, then you will become empty. This state will be easier to overpower. Some people start meditation and want to achieve things very quickly. They undermine this important concept and face dire consequences.

You must ensure that you are getting ample time to rest and have proper sleep. Lack of rest and sleep will make you weak. Your energy field will also get weak, and your protection cover will fade away.

Meditation is the art of relaxation. However, it is not a substitute for rest and sleep. You must give yourself an ample amount of time to remain fresh and rejuvenated. If you are facing a time crunch, then you should adjust your meditation time accordingly. It is not only the time of meditation practice that matters but your consistency, too.

You can practice at short intervals. Take some time out in the morning when you wake up. This is the best time to practice as your body is relaxed and your mind is fresh. It will also give a great kickstart to your day. In the evening, when you return from work, you can devote some time to meditation. This will help you in relaxing, and you will also sleep better.

Do not try to rush the process by overtaxing yourself in the beginning. It is a way of life that you will have to manage on a long-term basis. Finding a sustainable way to do it is always the best strategy.

Focusing on this simple aspect will help you in remaining steadfast, and it will also prevent you from the influence of negative energies.

A balanced diet

A simple fact of life is that we become what we eat. The food that we eat has a very strong influence on our lives. If you are eating an unbalanced diet, it will have a negative influence on your physical and mental wellbeing, as well as your spiritual consciousness. The activation of the third eye also gets heavily influenced by the kind of diet you have.

This is among the key reasons that the monks have very simple, yet healthy meals. They focus on supplying a healthy mix of macronutrients to their body. They eat the foods that can be easily processed by the body.

In this modern way of life where processed food has taken over the natural diet, it would be unwise to prescribe any strict eating regimen. However, you should stay away from an unbalanced diet. You must always eat the right mix of macronutrients that supply you with needed energy. Following diet plans or strict calorie control will expose you to negative energies as you become weak. It is a very unwise thing to do. You can also get the same results by having a diet that supplies all the required nutrients and eliminates the junk food that leads to excess weight. Whatever the diet plan you follow, you must ensure that it is nutritious.

Some people also get misled by the notion that fasting help in meditation. There is no doubt that fasting has a profound impact on meditation. It helps you in becoming calmer as the food always keeps reacting to your body and generates several kinds of reactions. However, fasting is only beneficial when it is done in a controlled manner. You cannot simply start fasting all of a sudden and expect positive results. In fact, the whole process would become counterproductive. Your mind will remain busy with the thoughts of food.

Fasting should only be done as a part of detoxification. It helps in cleaning your body of the toxic stuff and should not be over-stretched. Creating irregular gaps in your meal will only harm your efforts. Regular meals have a great role in reinforcing your astral body. You feel more content and vital.

You must focus on foods that have a lot of antioxidants and help in fighting free radicals. Eating easily digestible food is always the best way to remain healthy and fit. Complex foods, especially red meat, take a lot of time to digest. It also promotes the growth of negative energies in your body. You should try to avoid it as much as possible.

Remain joyful

Sorrow or grief are dark emotions. They attract negative energies a lot. Somewhere deep down there is a grudge building up. The development of positive energies becomes difficult in such a state. Happiness, laughter, and positivity, on the other hand, keep the dark energies at bay. You become strong and remain protected.

You must cultivate happiness. Try to remain cheerful. If you are unhappy about a few things in the past, try to forgive and forget them. Moving on will be easier for you. Moving on the path of third eye awakening with baggage from the past is not a healthy thing. Joy and peace are important in life. In fact, happiness has been the ultimate goal of the majority of people who have walked on this earth. Sadness and depression only weigh you down. Make your choice prudently.

Don't intoxicate yourself

The intoxication of any kind may give you a temporary relief from the problems of this world, but it cannot be a permanent solution. In fact, it isn't a solution at all. Problems generally become bigger when you come out of a hangover. You must stay away from avoid this scenario.

Drugs and alcohol have become quite popular. They cause hallucinations and make you see an imaginary world which you may like. However, they take you far away from reality.

Drugs and alcohol can be dangerous while you are on the path of third eye activation. You may hallucinate and have false visualizations. They also make you weak and incapable of exercising any control. You become weak and may become influenced by negative energies. You must stay away from them to remain protected.

Some Effective Ways to Manage Energies

Choose your colors wisely

The color you wear will have a profound impact on the amount of energy you absorb. Light colors do not absorb energy. This will help you a lot in staying safe from the influence of negative energies. This is one of the reasons white color is the preferred color for meditation. It reflects negative energies.

Dark colors attract and absorb energy. If you are wearing dark colors while doing your meditation, then the chances of coming in contact with the dark energies increase.

Find a positive place for meditation

The place of meditation has a very strong impact. A place with an excess of negative energies will always give you a hard time in meditation. You will be able to feel an intense pressure. There will be distractions and you will find it difficult to concentrate for long. If you find yourself in any such situation, then the chances are that you are sitting on a fault line. Shifting the place of meditation even by a few feet can make a lot of difference.

You can take remedial steps for correcting the flow of energy, yet fighting it for long will not yield great results. Shift the place of your meditation and find a corner that has a positive flow of energy or an energy well. Such a place will have a soothing impact and you will be able to meditate effortlessly.

Wash your hands

Once you start meditation, your sense of perception of the outside energy forces increases. You are able to feel their interaction with your body. You will be able to feel the extra pressure on your hands. You will become aware of energy building up around you. These realizations will become common. All this happens because you start attracting more energy toward yourself.

Whenever you feel any such pressure in your hands, you must wash them thoroughly under running water. It will increase your perception. It will also keep you safe from such energies.

Purify the room

The presence of negative and positive energies is beyond your control in any place. However, managing as best as you can is always in your interest. If you feel that your home or the place of meditation has a high concentration of negative energies, then you can take some proactive steps to balance these energies.

Burn incense or candles

Burning incense or candles have a positive impact on the energies. You can make the positive energies stronger by this method. It also helps in purifying the room. It gets filled with positivity and smells great. You will be able to meditate for longer.

Hot and cold treatment

Creating a temperature variation in the room is also a way to deal with the flow of energy. You can use heaters to make your room as warm as possible, and let it become cold afterward. Creating a temperature difference in the room helps immensely.

Get in sync with the lunar cycle

The moon has a deep impact on the energies on the

earth. It generates a great force. Even the oceans and currents do not remain unaffected by the influence of the moon. The behavior of energies varies on the full moon and new moon. You must consider this factor.

A full moon night is the best time to meditate. You will feel an explosion of energy during this period. It is a very suitable time for intellectual realization. The chances of third eye awakening are very high in this phase of the month. You must make the best use of this time.

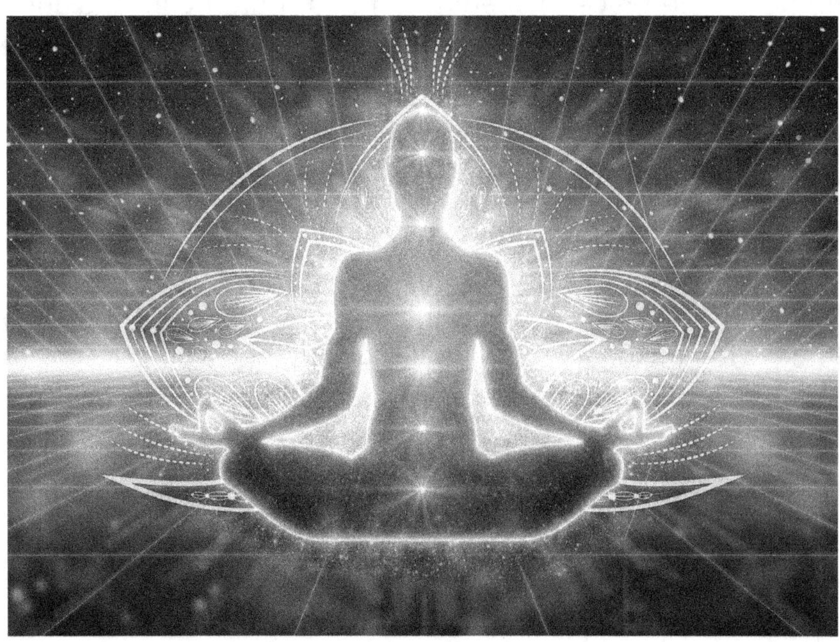

Chapter 21.
The Effect Oy Yoga
On Chakras

Everybody loves good health. More than anything, physical wellness contributes largely to our overall well-being. Therefore it is not surprising that people place a priority on their physical well-being. One of the many ways that people take care of their health is exercise. There are various other ways such as the constant intake of a balanced diet, lot of rest, frequent medical checkups and many more. Many find it easy to discipline themselves, their body and their appetite. This is done basically with the aim of keeping the body fit and healthy. One of these many ways of keeping the body fit is Yoga. Just like exercise or diet, Yoga is a combination of many different activities, and these activities are most effective when they are repeated again and again. The continuity enhances its effects in the body. Beyond exercise, yoga is not only targeted at the body but it is very important to the mind.

If over time, you have practiced yoga, beyond doubt, you

have experienced its benefits. It could be evident in your sleep, your health generally or your muscles and bones. It is quite easier to explain these benefits to an ardent believer in yoga, especially one who has practiced it time and over again. These same explanations may add complications to your discussion with someone who has never practiced yoga. Yoga has gone beyond a locally accepted practice and it is beginning to enjoy the attention it deserves from researchers. Scientists have started pinning down evidences on the effects of Yoga on health, how it works to ease pain and aches and most importantly, how it keeps the individual away from frequent hospital visits. These scientific explanations make it easier to draw more people to their mats. The practice of Yoga makes you more flexible, increases the strength of your muscles, perfects your posture, prevents cartilage and joint breakdown, increases your blood flow, increases your heart rate, drops your blood pressure and helps you establish a healthy lifestyle amongst other benefits.

Beyond the benefits of yoga to your body, there are other benefits that are more related to your mind and indeed, your overall well-being. Yoga helps you focus. This practice gives your mind room to relax, builds your inner strength, increases your self-esteem, and brings you into guidance. You would be learning from an expert, a yoga teacher who already has experiences and knows how best to employ yoga to your advantage. It also helps you build self-awareness and improves the quality of your relationships. Yoga helps you understand yourself better, this understanding is then extended to others.

There is no overemphasizing the numerous benefits of yoga, on your body, mind and relationships. You may be yet to determine if it is truly beneficial to all aspects of your body and life. Beyond doubt, it is. Yoga takes care of your body to the least of the details, including the chakras. How amazing is it that there is a single practice that can help you this much? If nothing has convinced you about yoga, let this do the work. Yoga does an amazing job on your chakras.

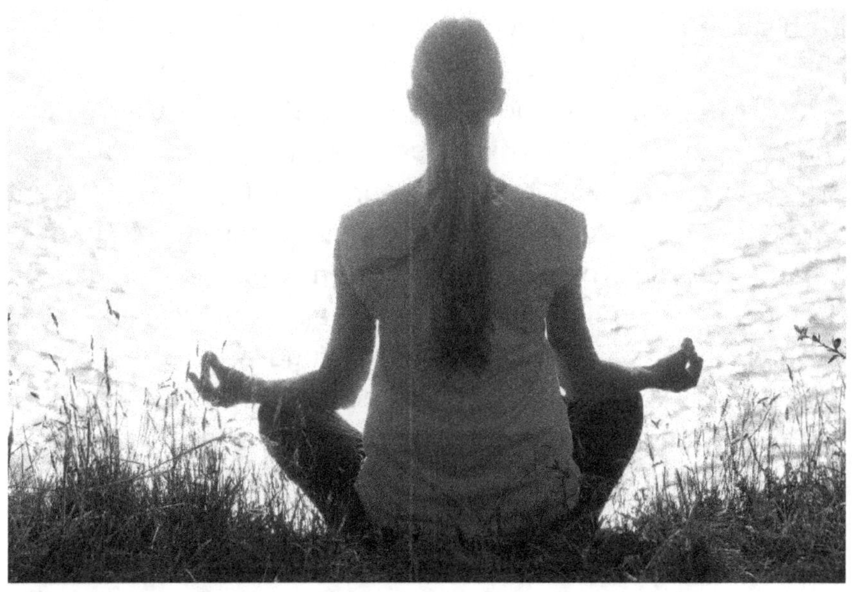

YOGA AND THE CHAKRAS

While you practice yoga, there is a life force energy that goes through the body within a number of channels. The life force energy is the 'prana ', while the series of channels are known as 'nadis. The channels are divided into parts at various points of amplified energy. These are the chakras. Each is responsible for certain responses to stimuli, certain values and behavior in our lives. Some of these life issues directed by the chakras include love and communication. There are other such issues. The chakras are also responsible for regulating different body systems, one of which is the skeletal system. Each chakra has a connection to a particular color along the rainbow, as well as a specific element, mantra.

It is possible for the series of channels to get blocked. When this happens, the chakras also stagnate. At this point, the life force reduces in pace. This can reduce the health of our body, mind and emotions. What yoga does in this event is to purify and re-energize the channels, the chakras. The life force then continues to flow freely. It is a fact that yoga is one of the easiest ways to put each chakra into balance. This is because it creates alignment in the body. As you balance your body through different yoga postures, your body begins to regain stability. This balance causes the chakras to align. This has effects on the sets of behavior you exhibit. It also makes unlearning obsolete habits and values easier. Yoga practices train us to channel our energies correctly, applying pressure where we should and releasing tension where necessary. This practice is particularly important to the chakra because they are responsible for many other issues relating to our total well-being.

Beyond the general effects of stretching and aligning the chakras, yoga improves the functionality of each chakra.

YOGA AND THE ROOT CHAKRA

The root chakra is responsible for your emotional stability. It helps you feel grounded and keeps you assured that you can cope with any situation that comes along your way. Surely, you do not want to go about without this kind of confidence. It is the root chakra that supplies this balance to your body. The serenity and satisfaction that comes from this balance is desirable. It is good for you and the people around you. Yoga helps you find this balance in your root chakra. This chakra is situated at the lowest part of the spine, the pelvic floor and the first three vertebrae. This chakra supplies the feeling of being deeply rooted in our lives.

It is all about finding balance. The root chakra acts as the balance base for the individual's body and life. You are not supposed to retain excess energy in this chakra and you also have to gather enough energy here. Your need to release and gain energy in the Muladhara is taken care of by yoga practices. Yoga helps you retain as much energy as you need in the root chakra. Realizing the fact that excess energy is bad for you, you can also shed the excess through yoga. The balance the yoga helps you achieve sets the ground for true transformation and personal growth in you. Some yoga postures that help you find balance in this region include Sukhasana, Balasana, Malasana, Uttanasana, Mountain pose, Sun salutations, Anjaneyasana, etc.

YOGA AND THE SACRAL CHAKRA

The sacral chakra located at the inner pelvis and lower belly helps the body to achieve flow, flexibility and fun. Here is where your relationship with yourself and other people is coordinated. Yoga opens up your chakra and this opening and alignment allow each chakra to operate at the best frequency. What would you do without the beautiful relationships in your life, what about the way you look into the mirror and you are totally in love with who you see? Do you know the amount of work it takes to understand yourself and the people around you?

You give yourself a better chance at these things as you practice yoga. The level of relaxation that yoga allows in your body and mind opens up this chakra and allows you to convert and harness the energy here to creativity and an amazing amount of understanding, first of yourself and then, other people. You gain a deeper understanding of your default reactions and emotions. Of course, the essence of self-awareness and healthy relationships cannot be over emphasized, as this is highly consequential to our mental health. When the sacral chakra is not aligned with others, some physical conditions can be visible. They include low back pain, urinary tract infections, impotence, ovarian cysts and some other reproductive issue.

Poses like Dvipada Pitham (bridge pose), Salamba Bhujangasana, (Sphinx pose), Kapotasana (pigeon pose), Dharunasana (Bow pose) as well as many other such poses will help you open up your sacral chakra. An open sacral chakra has significant effects on the overall health of an individual. .

YOGA AND THE THIRD CHAKRA

It is not unusual as we run through life, to come across certain individuals who do not have the least idea what to do in life, what they feel they should be doing or who they are meant to be. The Manipura, otherwise known as the navel chakra is responsible to provide answers to these questions of an individual. This chakra is directly connected to the sense of self. Other issues like identity, self-esteem, sense of purpose, individual will and personal identity are all associated with the sacral chakra. Digestion and metabolism are physical processes also dependent on the navel chakra. A misaligned navel chakra can easily make food impossible to digest.

Yoga keeps the chakra open, balanced and aligned. This opening allows you to get in touch with your inner being, your inner will and purpose. It is not rare to find that people who practice yoga have a certain cool around them that they have achieved over time. There is no other way to explain this than the word 'peace'. This sense of peace and purpose is enough to supply anyone with the energy needed to live a life that is both challenging and exciting.

Some of the poses you may want to try in order to open up your third chakra include Kapalabhati (breath of fire), Virabhadranasa III (Warrior III), Parivrtta, Trikonasana (Triangle pose), Parsvottanasa (Pyramid pose), and many others. These different poses are aimed at opening up your chakra and aligning it with other chakras.

YOGA AND YOUR ANHATA CHAKRA

No matter the day or time, matters of the heart are as important as life itself. Be it your physical body or the quality of your life, your heart has a whole lot of say in the matter. The importance of the heart to the body can never be over explained and its importance to life is just as grave. What would you do without a beating heart? Life is too beautiful to risk going through it with a heart closed up and tired. Good thing, there is a way to heal it. The fourth chakra, which happens to be the central point of the others, is the heart chakra.

The Anhata chakra is associated with compassion and unconditional love. It is from here that you come in contact with profound truths that you may never be able to explain to anybody else. It also serves as a bridge between the lower and the upper chakras. The way you align, open and heal your heart chakra is through the practice of Yoga. The yoga poses that are directed to this chakra open the area of the chest and they help to balance the heart chakra. Poses like Camel, Standing bow pose, Cow face pose force your chest to open. The science behind it is that your heart is located in the chest region. As your chest opens up, your heart chakra is aligned.

Opening your heart chakra removes restlessness, impatience, irritability, lack of trust and lack of empathy. All of which are capable of inhibiting you from enjoying healthy relationships with others as well as with yourself. These are all possibilities that you can attain through the constant practice of the yoga poses mentioned earlier. You can begin to experience how amazing it is to give and receive empathy, trust and love.

YOGA AND THE FIFTH CHAKRA

Vishudda chakra located at the throat is the purification center. Faith, expression, inspiration and communication are all controlled here. When this chakra is balanced, you can be sure of fluent and clear thoughts, creative written and spoken expression and wisdom. Opening up your fifth chakra through yoga is important to your well-being as a person and as a body. There are various symptoms that will be visible because of the deficiencies caused by a closed chakra. Some of them include headaches, hoarseness, sore throat, neck pain, and so on.

The symptoms can go beyond the physical to include the fear of speaking, shyness, stubbornness, social anxiety, inability to express thoughts and ideas, detachment, inhibited creativity. Nobody wants to go on unable to express their deepest thoughts and emotions, no one wants to go through life without the boldness it takes to stand up for our belief, stand up to people when it is necessary and get things done when we need them to be done by others. The throat chakra has to be balanced and open to help you achieve all that. Yoga becomes very important to us because it is one very certain way of improving fluency, clarity, creativity and wisdom.

There are different yoga poses for the throat chakra. Some of these poses are Matsyasana (Fish), Halasana (Plow), Salamba Sarvangasana (Supported Shoulderstand), King pigeon (Kapotasana), and many others. These poses allow you to stretch and exercise your neck, thyroid gland and head.

Yoga And The Sixth Chakra

Have you ever had a gut feeling about something or someone that you cannot explain? It was your third eye at work. Ajna, the sixth chakra is spectacular for perception. Often regarded as the third eye, it is responsible for controlling higher mental activities such as mental and emotional intelligence and insight. A properly aligned sixth chakra will come in handy the next time you need to make a business decision or any other important decision. A keen imagination, strong intuition and deep spiritual awareness are all resultant effects of a balanced and healthy third eye. This balance is not farfetched. You can ease yourself into it through the constant and consistent practice of yoga.

Some yoga poses that can help you activate this chakra include Child, Pyramid, Seated head to knee, side seated angle and so on.

Yoga And The Sahasrara Chakra

A certain connection with the universe is important for the individual. Have you ever felt disconnected from the entire universe? It is a feeling of despondence, lack of direction and a lack of self-understanding that results in the end. The crown chakra which happens to be the seventh helps you connect with the rest of the universe and its energy. This chakra also heightens your consciousness and pure wisdom. This is the point where the truth of the universe sits within us. Of course, you want your seventh chakra aligned, and balanced. A balanced Sahasrara results in bliss, intuitive knowledge and deeper understanding. Poses that are beneficial to your crown chakra are supported headstand, corpse pose, lotus pose, tree pose and some others.

Yoga is great for the body in a general sense, but the benefits this practice holds for the seven chakras is undeniable. If you have not added yoga to your list of frequent practices, it would be great to do that now. There is no denying the fact that yoga activates, balances, aligns and opens up your chakras.

Chapter 22.
Foods That Help
With Healing

Everyone knows that the foods you eat make a difference in the way you feel. All health specialists will tell you the same thing. However, did you know that certain foods can help to heal your chakras? They can, and it's worthwhile knowing the right kinds of foods to eat. You should also be aware that drinking sufficient water is also essential. Be mindful when you eat; chewing your food and enjoying all the tastes and textures, instead of eating on the go. Your digestive tract is the largest part of your body and if you don't give it the respect that it needs it can really give you problems – both physical and psychological. Thus, the chakras will be affected. Take your time and get used to using all of your senses actually to get more from your food. Start thinking of your food as being your friend, rather than simply the fuel you need to keep on living. There's a difference between simply living and actually optimizing your health and happiness.

You have probably heard in recent health articles about the benefits of eating brightly colored vegetables. That's certainly true when it comes to chakra healing. If you can incorporate red foods and beets into your diet, you will benefit, though don't overdo the beets as this may affect your throat chakra temporarily, taken in excess. Your root chakra is keen on spiced food, and a little tabasco sauce won't go amiss. You may even feel like your body craves this kind of taste. Learn to listen to it. It will serve you well to do so. You will also find that your root chakra enjoys lean meat, while your throat chakra is well served by a variety of fresh fruit or fruit juices. If you tend to be overweight and/or suffer from diabetes, avoid orange juice, as this concentration of fruit sugar may be detrimental to your health and fresh fruit would be a better option.

Your Solar Plexus Chakra will find its healing source in whole wheat bread, which will help in digestion. Healing can also be found in teas that are intended to calm the stomach, such as peppermint and chamomile. You may find that you enjoy eating peppermints, and rather than add the unnecessary sugar to your diet, a glass of peppermint tea is the preferred option. If you don't like drinking water, why not try adding a peppermint cordial to it, as this will also help you considerably.

Green tea is the tea of choice for the Heart Chakra, and this is particularly good for many health issues, so you won't be doing yourself a disservice introducing it as a regular drink to take the place of coffee or soda. Coffee and tea are stimulants and if you can cut down on the amount of them you drink, the better you will feel for it. The Crown chakra isn't a chakra that is affected by the foods that you eat. This is the chakra that prefers to have regular sunshine, relaxation, peace, and quiet. This chakra is calmed by meditation or relaxation exercises.

Diet in General

As a human being, you will be all too aware of your shortcomings when it comes to eating and drinking the right items. You know from normal health issues how food affects the way that you feel, but did you know how important water is to the body? Water helps to digest your food correctly, but it does much more than that. Water replenishes the body and the lost fluids that are needed for your movement and digestion. Water is especially important for those who suffer from ailments such as fibromyalgia or arthritic conditions who often forget that lack of movement and lack of water can make their situations worse. Make sure that you drink small amounts during the course of the day, which will help your chakras and will also help you to feel better.

If you know that you have been eating in excess and that this includes all of the wrong foods, one thing that can help you to detox is nettle tea. This is a wonderful way to make sure that your body keeps up its power to clean out all of the toxins that life has let get in the way.

There are many ways that you are able to work on the diet that you are taking in. Most Americans are on a diet that is not all that healthy or good for them. They are used to going out to eat all of the time, picking up something that is quick and easy at a local restaurant and using that to feed their families. This can cause a lot of bad stuff to happen to the body because all those bad nutrients, such as the sodium, the sugar, the bad fats, and the processed carbs, are all going to wreak some havoc on the body. And if the body is not able to get some of the nutrition that it needs, it is very hard for the chakras to work properly.

This means that it is time to work on making some changes to the diet that you are eating. If the description above seemed to fit into the lifestyle that you currently have, it is important to make the changes. The first changes to make is to get rid of the stuff that is so bad for the body. These are so unhealthy for the whole body and are just making you sick with all the added bad nutrients and calories.

In addition, you need to be careful about the bad sugars and sodium that are in your foods, as well as the fats and the carbs that you are taking in. Sometimes these are going to sneak their way into your diet so you need to become good at reading the labels before you purchase or make the meals for your family to eat. Watch out for some breads, some sauces, all baked goods, ice creams, French fries and more if you want to get rid of some of the bad foods that are in your diet.

Now it is time to move on to some of the foods that you should be eating to stay healthy. Here, you want to pick out foods that are healthy and whole. These are the foods that are so good for the body because they are able to provide the body with all the good nutrients that it needs, without having to put on all of the foods that are bad on the body and can make it sick. There are a few selections that you can go with including the following:

Lean meats: you will want to focus on the lean meats because they provide the body with some healthy protein that is so good for you and for helping your muscles to grow as strong as they need. While ground beef can work sometimes, but you will want to be careful because it can contain some more bad fats and cholesterol than your body needs. Lean meats like turkey, chicken, and fish are great because they provide all of the protein that the body needs without the bad stuff.

Healthy fruits and vegetables: make sure to add as many of these to your diet as you are able to each day. Fresh fruits and vegetables are so good for the body because they don't contain like any of the bad stuff that you need to worry about, they are low in calories, and you will be able to get a ton of the nutrients that you are looking for to keep the body nice and strong.

Healthy carbs: you do not have to avoid carbs all together, but you do need to be careful about the types of carbs that you are consuming. You do not want to focus on the processed and white carbs, such as those found in cheap breads or those in baked goods. These are basically going to be turned into sugars in the body which can raise your blood sugar levels and much more. Make sure that you stick with the varieties that are whole grain and will provide some added fiber and other nutrients to the diet you consume.

Low fat dairy: dairy is sometimes given a bad name, but it has a lot of the calcium that you need to keep the body nice and strong. This calcium, as well as vitamin D, can be great for the brain, the muscles, and so much more. You do need to be careful about the types of dairy that you consume. For example, if you have yogurt, you should make sure that you stick with a low fat plain yogurt and then add in fresh fruit if you would like to have that added flavor in there rather than going for the yogurt that already has the fruit inside.

In addition to making sure that you are eating the foods

that you should, you will want to make sure that you are preparing the food in the proper way. You should be making these meals at home and use approved cooking methods, such as baking and steaming, rather than frying. If you are someone who is always busy and on the run, you may want to consider working with some freezer meals. With a freezer meal, you would just spend a day or two putting together some meals and then they are ready in the freezer for you any time that you need. They do take a bit of prep work to get all put together, but the convenience of being able to grab a meal when you need it rather than wasting money and harming your body is so worth it.

When you are able to follow some of the tips above about dieting and eating a diet that is full of the healthy nutrients that you need to function and feel good, you are going to notice some huge changes in your chakras. Your body will feel good, so your chakras are able to function the way that they should. Give it a try and dedicate yourself to eating foods that are healthier than ever, and you are sure to notice that your chakras will feel better in no time as well.

Exercise

If you are taking yoga classes or practicing the yoga routines that we have mentioned in this book, then you will already understand that your body responds well to this kind of treatment. Couple that with the correct breathing methods and you begin to feel happier about your state of health and welfare. Your chakras need that exercise. They need your input to unblock them, and the silly thing is that most people do not understand the power they have actually to heal their lives. Once you begin this journey, you will find that you will never go back because you enjoy being who you are and have a better understanding of what your body is asking you to do. Yoga takes an individual and teaches that individual to understand the messages he receives from his body. The mind and body work together to form the perfect harmony needed to feel good about life. Think about and exercise your senses on a regular basis, as they will serve you well. Your sense of taste, smell, sight, and hearing are all tools to be used to make your life better. Don't neglect them and remember to be mindful of their needs.

Working out is something that most people do not want to spend their time on. They are worried that it is going to be too hard, they may feel bad that they aren't able to do some of the moves that are in the program, or they just don't want to put in the work. But the great benefits that you are able to get from working out on a regular basis are amazing, and these benefits are not all centered on losing weight or toning up, although those are nice as well.

It is important to find a good workout program to start right away to help your body feel as good as possible. There are a number of different workouts that you are able to do, and to help with your health it is best to work on them all together throughout the week. If you want to do some work with the chakras, though, it seems that yoga is one of the best options that you are able to choose from. This one will help you to work on your breathing techniques, will help to align the chakras a bit more, and can help you to feel amazing in no time.

In addition to working with yoga in your life, you may want to consider doing some of the other types of exercises to help the chakras feel a bit better. Working on cardio is a great way to get the heart up and working well, and can release some of the feel good emotions and the hormones that you need to feel happy and healthy. But while a lot of people are just going to focus on the cardio that they are able to do, it is important to spend some time on strength or weight training as well. This is a great way to make those muscles nice and lean without overdoing it and this helps to burn that metabolism a bit faster and get you on the right track to feeling amazing in no time.

And of course, spending some time with stretching is critical too, if you want to avoid causing injury to the whole body. This is where yoga and other forms of stretching can come into play and will make you feel more limber and ready to take on the things that are coming up in your life.

The trick to a good workout plan is to have a lot of variety so that you are able to work out a wide variety of muscles each day while not getting bored and wanting to give up. This is why you should try to find a way to mix together the cardio, the weight training, and the stretching throughout the week, so that you can work the different muscles, not end up harming something in the process, and you can continue to have some fun while you get in that good workout. Your mind, your body, and your chakras will all thank you for this hard work.

Chapter 23.
7 Signs That Your Chakras Are Out of Balance

Weight Problems

The chakras that are affected will be the sacral chakra, solar plexus chakra, and the root chakras. Most weight problems are considered to have lifestyle, dietary, or behavioral causes, along with exercise, but one cause the most people don't consider is not being grounded. If we don't feel grounded, this is a problem with the root chakra. If the root chakra is balanced, we will feel connected to nature. It won't matter what we might be facing in life; it makes us feel secure as all our basic necessities are being met. Most of us gain weight to help us feel grounded.

We might use weight as a buffer between the world and us when our self-esteem feels off or we feel intimidated or attacked. If this is the case, our solar plexus chakra might be unbalanced. The solar plexus chakra is our center of power. It helps with confidence, self-esteem, and control.

At times we have problems feeling pleasure and getting in touch with our emotions. If we bottle up feelings about what is happening around and in us and we don't process the emotions that might have shaped our feelings about survival and self-worth, we won't experience pleasure when we eat, and our sacral chakra becomes unbalanced.

If you have a severe problem with low body weight, an intense fear of gaining any weight, and your perception about your weight is distorted, you may have been diagnosed with anorexia. People who suffer from anorexia drastically restrict how much food they eat. Bulimia is when someone eats a huge amount of food and then either takes a laxative, makes himself or herself throw up, or exercises excessively. Both of these disorders will judge a person's appearance harshly because they think they have to be severely thin to be worthy. Individuals may have trouble controlling their own self-image because they think they have physical flaws. Both of these disorders are caused by an unbalanced solar plexus.

Mental Disorders

Anxiety: All of the chakras can be affected. It all depends on the type of anxiety you are experiencing. Anxiety is a part of our daily lives. When we get an intense, persistent, or excessive worry that takes over our existence, it is totally debilitating. If you suffer from anxiety, it could turn into terror or fear in minutes and, thus, turn anxiety into a panic attack. It can also mess up our quality of life.

It all depends on the type of anxiety you have, but it could affect any one of the chakras that are involved. If the crown chakra is out of balance, we might feel as if we aren't connected to the God, Goddess, Universe, Source, or Divine. If our anxiety is from the third eye being out of balance, we feel anxious about the unknown and we don't trust our intuition. You might feel anxious about saying how you actually feel, expressing yourself, and communicating with others if your throat chakra is not balanced. If are feeling intimidated, pressure to do well, completely overwhelmed by everything, or caught in a power struggle within a relationship, your solar plexus chakra is out of balance. If your sacral chakra is out of balance, you will have feelings of shame or guilt due to emotions that are so intense that you have not processed them completely. This can happen because of past traumas like sexual abuse. If we feel anxious about our surviving in this world like money, shelter, food, etc., the root chakra is not balanced. This makes us feel as if we are in a constant survival mode.

Depression: The chakras that are affected are the heart and crown chakras. Depression happens for many reasons. It might pass through temporarily at times. At other times, it could be a presence in our lives that never goes away. For people who suffer from depression, it could be debilitating. Depression might feel like constant hopelessness, emptiness, or sadness. You might not have any pleasure in your daily activities and feel like life isn't worth living. It might affect your sleep or appetite, causing you to sleep too much or not sleep at all. You might even have thought about suicide or death.

When you are depressed, you will have a deep-seated feeling of loneliness. If you feel connected to the world and the Universe, the crown chakra is balanced and open. If you feel angry toward the Universe about your life, this shows your energy is out of harmony. Having an unbalanced heart chakra might cause depression because we aren't connected to ourselves.

Panic Attacks: The chakras that are affected are the root, solar plexus, and heart chakras. Panic attacks happen when we are struck with disabling, acute, and sudden anxiety. These can be accompanied by feelings of impending doom, shortness of breath, shaking, trembling, sweating, increased heart rate, pounding heart, and palpitations. These attacks can happen if we aren't connected to our heart chakra and don't listen to what it is telling us. The root chakra gets involved when fear and panic set in since our fear for survival gets triggered. If our heart chakra feels disconnected and we are in a constant state of fear, the solar plexus feels as if we have been punched in the stomach since our confidence and self-esteem live here.

Cancer

All the chakras are affected by this horrible disease. Cancer happens when cells that are abnormal get created and divide at an uncontrollable rate. They infiltrate and destroy good body tissue. This can happen on many levels and symptoms can vary depending on the part of the body that gets affected. Symptoms might include thick areas under the skin, palpable lumps, skin changes, weight changes, fatigue, and many others. Factors that can increase the risk of cancer can include environment, health conditions, family history, habits, and age. The Mayo Clinic has stated that most cancers happen in people who don't have any known risk factors. Cancer could be the result of deep hurt and resentment that has not been processed, denied, or ignored. It can manifest in toxic emotions, grief, or hatred that eats away at us.

These manifest on several levels because of a result of having an imbalance in certain chakras:

- Cancers of esophagus, larynx, and thyroid: Throat chakra

- Lung cancer: Heart and throat chakras

- Brain tumors: Crown chakra

- Rectal and prostate cancer: Root and sacral chakra

- Cancers of rectum, colon, uterus, ovaries, and cervix: Sacral chakra

- Cancers of the pancreas, intestines, liver, and stomach: Solar plexus chakra

- Breast cancer: Heart chakra

Headaches

The chakras that are affected by this are the crown and third eye chakras. If you get headaches that aren't caused by physical imbalances, it might be an indication that one of your chakras is unbalanced. If you have a headache in the front that includes symptoms of pressure behind the eyes or sinus pressure, this is usually disharmony in the third eye.

This type of headache might indicate that you have been focusing on your intelligence and you fear your spirituality. You can only see the reality in life, and you don't trust your intuition. When these headaches happen, it is because you are ignoring the inner wisdom that you possess. If you get "hints" but never act on them, you aren't honoring your third eye's wisdom. You might feel like you need to pursue new opportunities, but you don't do so. You might also experience a knowing that a specific person might be ill and won't feel like being around others. You engage them anyway. Opposing intuitive hints could cause imbalance and discord with the third eye chakra.

If you have a headache on the top of your head in the center, it might be from an imbalance in the crown chakra. This might mean you have a hard time trusting your life path, or seeing the larger picture, or even finding faith in yourself and your connection to the Divine. You might also feel unsatisfied or alone.

Reproductive Issues

Infertility: The chakras that are affected by this will be the solar plexus, root, and sacral chakras. If a woman can't conceive a child after many attempts for over one year, this is called infertility. Many will experience infertility, but the fear, and frustration that the woman experiences creates a lot of stress and possibly shame. The sacral chakra is the one that is affected because it is associated with the genitals and womb and because it is the seat of all emotions. Most people who deal with infertility battle with many severe emotions. It makes them wonder, "Am I making the right decision?" "Do I even want to be a parent?" "Do I have the right partner?" "I might not even be a good parent." "How is this going to change my life?"

There could be physical causes like high follicle-stimulating hormone, lack of menstruation, low sperm count, poor egg quality, and other issues could be to blame. Most of the time, there is a high stress level for the people who are trying to conceive. Since infertility can trigger family issues, the root chakra is involved, too. For people who are trying to conceive, added difficulty can develop if they are trying to have a family and aren't getting any support from a significant other. They might also be worried about passing on undesirable traits to their children. Making a new life is a challenge to a person's self-esteem, it can make them feel powerless and this becomes a solar plexus issue since this is our power center.

Uterine Cysts and Fibroids: The chakra that is affected is the sacral chakra. The Mayo Clinic states that uterine fibroids are growths that are in the uterus that aren't cancerous. They often happen during childbearing years. A lot of women may experience uterine fibroids sometime in their lives. Most of the time, they don't cause any symptoms but for others, they can grow to a large size and cause pain during menstruation, when having a bowel movement, or when you are digesting food. They can cause problems in breathing.

Cysts are sacs filled with fluid that are located on the ovaries. If there is a growth inside the uterus, it might be a sign that the sacral chakra is not balanced. There is an actual block to the reproductive area. The energy is telling you that there is a blocked energy flow inside. You might be holding onto toxic, negative, and old thoughts, feelings, or emotions that are attempting to flow energy into dead ends. This could include relationships or jobs that you have outgrown or conflict with your relationships, reproduction, abundance, or creativity.

Joint Pain

Hip Pain: If you have problems with your hips that aren't caused by any physical trauma, there is usually a sacral chakra problem. Our hips hold onto a lot of unexpressed emotions that haven't been dealt with and that we keep avoiding. Since the sacral chakra is the seat of our emotions, we could cause an imbalance if we don't honor our feeling.

Leg Pain: The chakras that are affected will be the solar plexus or root chakra. Leg pain is usually linked to an imbalance in the root chakra. Leg pain might symbolize a resistance to moving forward in life. This could manifest in self-sabotaging behaviors that are based on fear, for example, a fear of failure or fear that we might not get what we want. If this is the case, the root chakra could be linked to the solar plexus chakra and both are out of balance. It is mainly a root chakra problem because of fear about clothing, water, food, housing, or bills.

Neck Pain: The chakra that is affected here is the throat chakra. If the neck pain hasn't been caused by any physical trauma, it could be that your throat chakra is out of balance due to the way you are interacting with the world. If you don't express yourself honestly and openly or if you try to hide specific parts of yourself like insecurities or fears from others, it can create imbalances to the throat chakra. There are many reasons why you might hold yourself back, but the end result is always the same: neck pain.

Sciatica: The chakra that is affected by this is the sacral and root chakras. Sciatica is pain that goes from the lower back down through the hips, buttocks, and down each leg. If it isn't caused by trauma, sciatic pain could mean a root chakra that is out of balance. This chakra deals with problems regarding your being and survival. If a primal problem comes up in your life: fear that your basic necessities will be taken away, whether or not you can provide for your children, how you will pay your bills, or if you be able to eat today, this means your root chakra is out of balance. Sciatica usually symbolizes your fear about the future and money. At times, if you have sciatic pain, it could mean you don't feel safe.

Back Pain: If you have pain anywhere in the back that wasn't caused by physical trauma, it might be telling you about your chakra health. Pain could range from a dull ache that makes your back tight to a sharp acute pain that hinders your range of motion.

Upper Back: The chakras that are affected are the heart and throat chakras. If you don't speak the truth or if you experience heartbreak, threats to loving yourselves or problems loving others, the tension could manifest as pain or tension in the upper back. You might feel as if you are holding back love, unloved, or unsupported.

Middle Back: The chakras that are affected are the solar plexus and heart chakras. Everyone has issues about love, holding onto hurts from the past, our power being challenged, or feeling loved, you might feel pain or tension in the middle part of your back. This might happen if you get stuck in those feelings from the past and might become filled with guilt over things you said or done.

Lower Back: The chakras that are affected are the root and sacral chakras. If you are feeling challenged in creative expression, relationships, or abundance, you might feel pain and tension in your lower back. Holding these emotions back or just not processing them and having problems with survival and getting your basic needs met might mean pain for your back.

Asthma and Allergies

The chakra that is affected is the heart chakra. If you experience narrow airways and are producing excess mucous, it could trigger shortness of breath, wheezing, and coughing. If you have allergies, your immune system will make antibodies that recognize a certain allergen is harmful, even if it isn't. Both of these conditions cause problems with one's daily life. Sometimes these conditions can be caused by a compromised immune system and might cause inflammation of your digestive system, sinuses, airway, or skin. It could also cause respiratory distress. Since these are in the heart chakra, such reactions might mean that this chakra is out of balance, especially if you have problems with compassion, love, heartache, and grief.

Chapter 24.
Chakras, Endocrine System And The Immune System

In addition to the benefits mentioned earlier, there are many things that chakras control including the efficient functioning of our endocrine system and our emotions. Let us look at each in a bit of detail:

Let us start by recalling the 7 primary chakras and their locations:

Root Chakra – situated at the base of the spine

Sacral Chakra – situated below the navel

Solar Plexus Chakra – situated above the navel

Heart Chakra – situated in the middle of the chest

Throat Chakra – situated in the throat

Third Eye Chakra – situated at the center of the forehead

Crown Chakra – situated at the top of the head

The Endocrine System

Next, let us look at the Endocrine System in our body. The Endocrine System is our body's central mechanism of control. It consists of many ductless glands that are responsible for secreting, producing, and distributing different kinds of hormones required for various physiological functions of our body.

These hormones are directly sent through the bloodstream to the places that need them. Effective functioning of the Endocrine System is essential for overall good physical and mental health. The Endocrine System consists of the following elements:

The Pineal Gland – The most important hormone secreted by this gland is melatonin that is responsible for maintaining and regulating your body's circadian rhythm or the internal biological clock. This cone-shaped gland along with the pituitary gland regulates and balances the entire biological and glandular functioning in our body. The third eye chakra can be activated optimally when the pineal and the pituitary glands work perfectly in tandem.

The Pituitary Gland – Also referred to as the 'master gland,' the pituitary gland controls the activities and functioning of most other glands. Attached to the hypothalamus (between the eyes), the pituitary gland regulates the functioning of other organs and other glands. It communicates via signals in different forms.

This pea-shaped gland works in tandem with the pineal gland controls and balances the overall smooth functioning of our body's physiological and biological activities. The energy of the third eye chakra can be released when these two glands are well synchronized with each other.

Pancreas – The two kinds of hormones produced by the pancreas are needed for two basic functions; one to aid in digestion and the other to control energy levels in our body.

Ovaries – These glands produce the female hormones namely progesterone and estrogen and also produce and release eggs for reproduction

Testes – These glands come in pairs and are responsible for the production and release of the male hormone, testosterone. They also produce and release sperms.

Thyroid – A very important gland, the thyroid is responsible for regulating the heart rate, the metabolic rate and also controls a few digestive functions along with bone maintenance, muscle control, and brain development. The thyroxin produced by the thyroid controls the rate at which our body converts stored food into energy for use. A malfunctioning thyroid can be quite a debilitating factor that comes in the way of a leading a happy life for anyone.

Parathyroid – This gland controls calcium levels in the bloodstream so that the muscles and the nerves function smoothly. The parathyroid also helps in keeping bones healthy and strong.

Hypothalamus – This gland responds to multiple external and internal factors and triggers various reactions to enable stability and a consistent state in our body. The hypothalamus triggers various physiological reactions in response to feelings of hunger, the temperature of your body, feelings of excessive eating, blood pressure, and others. Based on these conditions, it sends signals to other glands and organs to respond appropriately to these triggers to enable a stable and consistent condition of your body.

Adrenal Glands – These glands secrete different kinds of hormones referred to as 'chemical messengers' which travel through the bloodstream to triggers physiological and chemical reactions in various organs.

The Immune System

Millions and millions of cells come together and waltz together in perfect harmony exchanging critical information thereby triggering appropriate and important physiological, biological, and chemical reactions in our body. The cells of the immune system help organs and organ systems in our body to function smoothly helping us live a happy and peaceful life.

Moreover, those cells that are not performing optimally are retired and new ones are automatically generated to take their place thereby enhancing our health and our longevity. If these weak cells are not correctly replaced in the immune system, they end up sending erroneous signals to all parts of the body resulting in disorders and discomforts such as weak digestion, general body weakness and delayed recovery from even simple illnesses.

The way modern medicines work to set this right is by suppressing the action of the well-functioning cells too until such time all the cells do not achieve the same level of functioning. The medication is continued until all the cells in the immune system get back into the synchronized dancing pattern. This is where chakra healing can help in getting our immune system in order.

The Thymus Gland – It plays an important role in the production of T-cells which form an essential part of the white blood cells that form the core of our immune system. In fact, if you speak to any chakra healer, he or she will tell you the dance of the immune system is the most beautiful and well-coordinated dance in our body.

Chakras And Glands

If you notice the locations of the glands, you will see that they are more or less placed close to different chakras. Although the traditional systems do not speak about the connection between chakras and glands, the modern followers and experts started outlining clear connections between the various chakras, glands, organs and the immune system of the body.

Each chakra is connected to different glands of the endocrine system and facilitates the smooth functioning of that particular gland. Here is a list of the various chakras, the glands they regulate, their functions and the signs of warnings associated with an inefficiently functioning gland/chakra:

Root Chakra – This is connected to the adrenal glands and stands for self-preservation and physical energy. The issues that the root chakra and the adrenal glands handle are associated with survival and security. In the males, the sacral chakra is closely linked to the gonads. The fight/flight response of the adrenal glands located at the top of the kidneys is directly connected to the survival drive of the root chakra.

A weak root chakra could result in a weakened

metabolism and immune system resulting from a compromised working of the adrenal glands which are responsible for releasing and producing chemical messengers needed for all the physiological, chemical and biological functions of your body.

A not-so-strong root chakra results in nervousness and a sense of insecurity whereas an overly working root chakra could result in greed and a sense of excessive materialism.

Sacral Chakra – Governs the reproductive glands which are the ovaries (for the females) and the testes (for the males. The well-balanced and healthy root chakra facilitates the uninterrupted functioning of these glands ensuring well-developed sexuality in the person.

The root chakra also regulates the production and secretion of the sex hormones. The potential for life formation in the ovaries is reflected in the sacral chakra as these two energies are connected.

When this chakra is open and free, you are able to express your sexuality well without being overly emotional. You feel a comforting sense of intimacy with your partner. A healthy sacral chakra enhances your passion and liveliness and helps you manage your sexuality without feeling burdened with undue emotions.

A sacral chakra that is not functioning at its peak efficiency is bound to leave you frigid, very close to people and relationships, and poker-faced. On the contrary, a weak sacral chakra will make you feel overly and unnecessarily, emotionally compelling you to attach yourself to people for a sense of security and belonging. Your feelings could be overly sexual towards one and all.

Solar Plexus Chakra – This controls the pancreas, which is directly connected to the sugar (through the control of insulin secretion) and, therefore, energy levels in your body. Thus, if this chakra is not working properly you could potentially have a weak pancreas, resulting in a compromised metabolic state. Compromised pancreas could lead to digestive problems, lowered blood sugar levels, ulcers, poor memory, etc. which are all connected with a bad metabolism.

Heart Chakra – Regulates the thymus gland and through it, the entire immune system. Being the center of love, compassion, spirituality, and group consciousness, a malfunctioning heart chakra will result in the malfunctioning of the thymus gland leaving you prone to low immunity.

Our feelings and thoughts towards ourselves play a crucial role in keeping our immune system working well. When we love ourselves our immune system is powerful and strong. When we are uncertain of ourselves and our strengths and our capabilities, we feel disappointed which drives us to react wrongly to negative things.

All these negativities leave our immune system weak and we end up holding on to toxins. It is imperative to keep our heart chakra healthy by investing time and energy in self-love so that our immune system is strengthened. An underactive heart chakra makes you feel distant and cold and an overactive one could result in selfish love in your heart. Be wary of both states and work at keeping your chakra balanced.

Throat Chakra – controls and regulates the thyroid gland and hence is directly responsible for a healthy metabolism and to regulate body temperature. This is the center of communication and plays a vital role in the way you speak, write, or think. An unbalanced throat chakra results in a malfunctioning thyroid resulting in an overall poor physical, mental, and emotional health.

Third Eye Chakra – directly controls the functioning of the pituitary gland or the master gland which controls and regulates other organs and glands in the human body. The Pineal gland is many times associated with this chakra too, as we already know that a well-coordinated, combined working of the pineal and the pituitary glands is responsible to keep our entire body, mind, and spirit well-oiled and working well.

Crown Chakra – This regulates the functioning of the pineal gland, which controls our biological cycle and our circadian rhythm.

Connection Between Glands And Chakras

Even the slightest disturbances in the chakras or our energy centers can result in physical manifestations of issues and problems. When the chakras don't function efficiently the corresponding glands and organs they are associated with are also affected.

Chakras as you already know are the energy centers in our body and have no physiological or physical shape or form. These energy centers influence the way we live in different layers of our lives, including the biological, the physical, the emotional, and the psychic layers.

When any of the energy centers malfunction or become imbalanced, the problems are manifested in a physical, mental, or spiritual form. An underactive or an overactive chakra can cause problems for you. Keeping them balanced is critical for your overall health.

Any disturbance even in one energy center could result in problems in any other chakra and/or related glands and organs. For example, if there is a blockage in the heart chakra, you are going to feel unloved or listless or could have high blood pressure etc. All these problems could affect other organs which, in turn, can potentially harm associated chakras.

Therefore, it is imperative to keep all chakras in perfect balance to achieve overall physical, emotional, and spiritual health for yourself. Let us look at some examples of how a malfunctioning of chakras can affect the associated gland.

The Third Eye Chakra And The Pituitary And The Pineal Glands

When the third eye chakra is imbalanced or not working at its peak of efficiency, the functioning of both the pineal and pituitary glands will be affected leading to associated problems. For example, the pituitary is the master gland that regulates the functioning of other glands. So, when the third eye chakra is inefficient, other glands can also be affected negatively resulting in an overall breakdown of your systems.

The pituitary gland regulates intellect and emotion and working in conjunction with the pineal gland helps achieve overall balance in your body. The pineal gland will either resonate or counter the effects of pituitary gland for optimum benefit to our body and mind. Therefore, the third eye chakra is required to be given a lot of importance during your chakra healing and maintenance process.

The Heart Chakra And The Thymus Gland

Located in the middle of your chest, the heart chakra or the anahata controls and regulates the working of the thymus gland which is an important aspect of our immune system. A calm and balanced heart chakra results in an effectively-working nervous system and prevents undue agitation of your mind.

Here is a simple technique to help connect and activate your thymus gland. Tap gently in the middle of your chest at the collarbone level with your fingers. This helps in calming down agitated nerves. When you gently tap at the collar level about 3-4 inches away on each side helps to increase your energy levels.

Glands And Chakra Healing

Chakra healing will lead to improved functioning of the endocrine system which is great for physical healing of your body. The connection between glands and chakras represent a link between the energy points in your body to the physiological and physical functions.

Another useful entry point for chakra healing is the nervous system which is connected to glands and organs in multiple ways and at multiple points. A chakra healing session is ideally begun by calming the nerves and then targeting a particular gland and/or chakra.

By understanding the connection between chakras and the glands, you can use healing in different ways that will help you overcome physical, emotional, mental, and spiritual issues in your body and mind. Connecting the chakras and the glands will help in your overall well-being.

Chapter 25.
The Science Behind Chakras

When you hear talk about chakras the first thing you associate them with is probably spirituality. After all, the concept of chakras has its roots in ancient India, the very personification of spirituality if there ever was one! From Hindu gods and goddesses to the origins of Buddhism, ancient India covers a wider spectrum of spirituality and religious tradition than just about any other place or culture on the face of the Earth. Modern-day forms of meditation and yoga owe their very existence to the mystics and healers of the subcontinent. Therefore, it is no wonder that the tradition of chakras evokes such a rich and reverent sense of spirituality. However, there is another side to chakras, one which is more modern and certainly less spiritual, at least at face value. This other side is the science behind chakras.

Modern science has produced countless discoveries in

terms of the human body and the role that energy plays in our very existence. While the concept of energy is certainly nothing new, the quantification of energy definitely is. Never before have we been able to actually see and measure the amounts of energy being generated by a living thing. With today's science and technology such feats are now commonplace. In fact, much of modern medicine utilizes the ability to measure and monitor the energy levels within the human body, thus determining the health and wellbeing of an individual in ways that the ancient mystics of India would have doubtlessly understood all too well. After all, the idea that energy makes up all living things is something we might consider revolutionary in scientific terms, but it is very old news to those who have been practicing chakra health and wellbeing. Indeed, the knowledge that we have obtained through modern breakthroughs in technology has done little more than validating the ancient traditions of chakra energy and their role in human life.

One of the first things to recognize when it comes to the science behind chakras is the significance of just where the chakras are located. Placing the energy centers of the subtle body along a central axis makes good sense as they are more balanced and centered along that line. However, you could ask why chakras weren't placed below the Root Chakra position, at the knees or feet for example. Alternatively, you could question why chakras were not allocated to the hands. After all, what part of the body is more associated with energy than the hands or the feet? Yet the seven main chakras are contained within a short span, traveling up the central axis of the human body along the spinal column. And here is where the science behind chakras begins to take shape. It turns out that the spinal column is, in fact, the conduit through which electrical impulses are transmitted from the brain to all other parts of the body. The nerves which run through the spinal column are virtual telephone lines, bringing every sort of message from the command center of the brain to all other parts of the physical body. Thus, the spinal column is nothing short of an energy highway, seeing energy flow from the brain to the body and from the body back to the brain again.

The fact that the spinal column is the path for energy to flow throughout the body would be enough to get anyone to consider the validity of the chakras, regardless of their spiritual beliefs. However, this is not the end of the story. What is even more striking is that the locations of the lower five chakras correspond directly to actual nerve clusters along the spinal column. This means that not only did the ancients understand the function of the spinal column, but they also were aware of the significance of the nerve clusters along it! Just as the chakras are considered energy centers of the subtle body, the nerve clusters along the spinal column, five in total, are actually energy centers of the physical body. Some might argue that this is nothing spectacular. After all, if anyone studied a dissected body, they would see the nerve centers in the spinal column. While this is true, it must be understood that those same ancients had no modern equipment with which to measure the energy in those nerve centers. Thus, those nerves could have served any function to the casual observer. Yet the ancient Indian sages knew somehow that those bundles of nerves were, in fact, the centers of energy in the physical human body.

Perhaps this is a classic matter of which came first, the chicken or the egg? While it is possible that the ancients studied the anatomy of the body, it is also entirely feasible that their knowledge of the chakras had little or nothing to do with their understanding of the human body. We may never know what inspired their belief in seven separate energy centers along a central axis, but what we can be sure of is that their knowledge goes hand in hand with the knowledge we are only now beginning to acquire regarding how the physical body works. It is therefore entirely possible that the ancients were made aware of the workings of the subtle body and that only now can we see the direct correlation between our subtle form and our physical form. Either way, modern science, and medicine have only served to validate the concept that energy centers do in fact exist along the spinal column, and that the health and wellbeing of these centers greatly impact our overall physical health and wellbeing.

The five nerve clusters along the spinal column account for the first five chakras, beginning with the Root Chakra and ending with the Throat Chakra. While the Third Eye Chakra and the Crown Chakra are not located in the spinal column itself they still follow the same central axis. There are a few theories regarding the scientific nature of these two chakras, and it is worth examining two of the main ones. First, there is the theory that the sixth and seventh chakras are related to the pineal and the pituitary glands. In the case of the sixth or the Third Eye Chakra, the pineal gland is seen as the corresponding energy center. The significance of this is that the pineal gland is responsible for creating melatonin which regulates sleep patterns. Since the third eye is considered the subconscious mind in many traditions it is profoundly significant that the Third Eye Chakra would be located in a place where sleep, and thus dreams are regulated. Many ancient traditions view dreams as the realm of the subconscious, equally real and important to physical reality. The idea that the ancients placed the seat of the intellect and subconscious mind in the same vicinity as the pineal gland has to be far more than mere coincidence.

Physicians and philosophers alike have attributed the pineal gland with such things as the intellect and even the soul itself. René Descartes was a world-renowned scientist and philosopher in the sixteen hundreds. He wrote several books on anatomy and the soul, two of which dealt with the pineal gland in particular. According to Descartes, the pineal gland was where our soul resided and was the very place where all thoughts originated. While modern science is still struggling to understand the complexities of the human brain it might be time to consider the patterns already emerging. The fact that the pineal gland is responsible for sleep, and thus dreams, and that some prominent thinkers have attributed it to the center of thought and the subconscious self, coupled with the fact that the Third Eye Chakra is located in the same region, should be enough to convince anyone that these assertions are in fact true. Again, this is just one more example of where the physical body closely mirrors the dynamics of the subtle body.

The Crown Chakra, or the seventh chakra, is the highest chakra of the seven. Located at the crown of the head, it resides between the physical body and the realm beyond. One theory links this chakra with the pituitary gland, which makes a lot of sense when you understand the functions of the pituitary gland. The main function of the pituitary gland is to produce and secrete hormones—chemicals that affect functions throughout the rest of the body. Some of the functions affected by the hormones produced by the pituitary gland include Thyroid function, water absorption, and regulation of temperature, pain and pain relief, regulation of blood pressure, growth, and sex organ functions. All in all, the pituitary gland can be seen as a controller of just about every facet of the physical body's function and wellbeing. In a way, the pituitary gland is like the conductor of an orchestra, overseeing that every member of the orchestra performs their part exactly as it ought to be performed. Is it any wonder that this is where the chakra associated with a higher being is located? After all, what function does the Higher Being have than to oversee and regulate the function of all life? Again, is its mere coincidence that the chakra centers have been placed where they have, or is modern science simply revealing that the wisdom of the ancients is, in fact, accurate and deserves greater attention and respect?

The association of the sixth and seventh chakras with the pineal and pituitary glands is just one theory which serves to confirm the validity of the chakra tradition. Another theory which deserves attention is the one that focuses on the general regions of the Third Eye and Crown Chakras. This theory doesn't focus on specific glands, but rather it focuses on the area of the brain and the top of the head. In the case of the sixth or Third Eye Chakra, the location of this chakra is basically in the forehead region, which is where the brain itself is largely located. Again, this has great significance as the brain is scientifically known to be the seat of all thought, emotions and even dreams, thus it can be considered the seat of the subconscious. While this is nothing new in terms of our understanding of the human condition, it should be noted that different cultures throughout history viewed things quite differently. The ancient Greeks, for example, saw various organs as the seat of the soul, including the heart, liver and even the abdomen. In fact, the Greeks believed that the lower organs were the originators of emotional joy and or pain.

That said, the notion that the brain is the center of thought, creativity, and even the subconscious is, in fact, a very recent one. Only within the last few hundred years has the seat of the mind found its way to the head. Thus, the fact that the ancient Indian sages placed the chakra responsible for intellect and wisdom in the forehead was far more than mere luck. Again, due to the primitive science and technology available at the time it is hard to imagine that the placement of the Third Eye Chakra had anything to do with a deeper understanding of human anatomy and physiology. Rather, it seems that by understanding the workings and design of a person's subtle body the ancients were able to lay the foundations for a more accurate and in-depth understanding of the workings and design of the physical body.

The Crown Chakra is a bit of a mystery in terms of its location on the human body. Depending on the tradition you read, this chakra is located at or just above the crown of a person's head. In terms of spiritual significance, this makes perfect sense as the Crown Chakra is literally your connection to the higher realm of spirit. In a sense you could relate the Crown Chakra to the leaves on a tree, existing between the tree itself and the air all around it. And, just as the leaves of a tree absorb the energy from the air and the sun, so too, the Crown Chakra absorbs the energy from the higher realms. Still, this doesn't really do much for proving that the ancients had some advanced understanding of how the physical body worked as a result of their insights regarding the subtle body. That is unless you consider a concept that is gaining more and more acceptance within the scientific community. This concept is the one regarding auras. The aura of a person is literally an envelope of energy that radiates from and surrounds the person. Recent advances in photographic and electromagnetic technology have enabled us to actually see the human aura for the first time in recorded history. And this phenomenon has gone a long way to changing our understanding of how energy affects life overall.

While a person's aura envelops their whole body, the most visible elements of it are around the head. Thus, the virtual energy of a person can be seen just above their shoulders and above the crown of their head. This is where the ancient symbol of the halo comes to mind. When we think of a halo we are reminded of the holiest people, or angels or deities themselves. Additionally, while halos are normally associated with Christianity, the fact of the matter is that they have representations throughout many traditions across many different times and places throughout history. Thus, while the traditions themselves may differ, the association of halos with purity or divinity remains constant. Furthermore, the more divine or holy a person was, the larger and brighter their halo was. Suddenly we have our physical connection with the location of the seventh chakra. The Crown Chakra—that which connects a person with the divine, is in the same place as the energy 'crown' of a person's physical body. And, just as this energy crown lingers on and just above the head, so too the Crown Chakra does the same. Due to the realization that our physical body has an energy envelope of sorts, our representation of the human form may have to be changed from its current physical only form to one which incorporates its energy aspect as well.

The fact that modern science has discovered energy centers in the same locations as for where the ancients placed the seven main chakras is nothing short of extraordinary. Even the harshest skeptic would have to take a moment to consider the significance of what this actually means. However, in case you thought that this was the only correlation between the chakra traditions and modern science, rest assured, there is more! The chakras and the nerve centers are described as focal points for energy. This energy was seen as the electrical communications between the brain and the body and nothing more for many years. However, modern breakthroughs in the fields of electromagnetism and quantum physics have led to yet more correlations between modern science and ancient wisdom. Modern research has begun to determine that not all energy is the same. Just as radio waves exist on different frequencies, so too, energy can exist in different forms. The variations of energy are often referred to in terms of vibrations. Lower vibrations create different forms of energy than higher vibrations. In fact, it is theorized that matter itself is merely energy on a really low vibrational frequency. This is the basis of all teleportation theories. Converting matter to energy is not as difficult as it once seemed since matter itself is now seen as a level of energy. Still, how does this relate to chakras? Simply put, science is now realizing that the human body does, in fact, absorb energy from its surroundings as well as from the food that it ingests.

Once science realized that electromagnetic energy is all around us, moving past us and even through us at all times, the question was raised as to how this energy affected us. On the physiological level, certain energies can, in fact, be dangerous. People who live or work near areas with high electromagnetic activity often contract cancers and other ailments, now being linked to the high concentrations of energy. There has also been an association of energy and mood, suggesting that a person's mind can be directly influenced by the energy in the environment. At first, this doesn't make sense since energy, like radio waves, needs a receiver in order to be of any actual value. And, just like a radio, the human body would need to convert the energy received into usable information. Simply receiving the radio waves is not enough for a radio to play music. A radio must convert those radio waves back into vibrations in order to produce the appropriate sounds. Here we find two distinct correlations to chakra energy and wellbeing.

The first correlation is in terms of the chakras acting as energy centers. By understanding that energy flows around us and through us at all times, these centers take on a whole new meaning. Not only do they generate energy that flows through our physical and subtle bodies, affecting our overall health and wellbeing, but they also receive energy from the environment. This means that they absorb as well as generate energy. Thus, when a chakra is closed or damaged its ability to absorb useful energy is significantly reduced. This is like not being able to digest food properly. It is no wonder, in light of this, that damaged chakras can so significantly reduce a person's health and wellbeing. The importance of having healthy, vibrant chakras is therefore even more critical as the health of our chakras determines our ability to take in energy.

Chapter 26.
Things to Avoid

We can all get a little carried away in a practice or a process. We can get lazy and not put in as much effort as we should. There are always fluctuations with life because we need to be flexible when the unexpected occurs. When you are going through a chakra awakening experience it will be very 'eye-opening' and transformative. As a lot of people are discovering these tools and methods and choosing to align with higher consciousness, there are several reports available of what many people have encountered in their own experiences.

For a lot of us, it is an amazing and powerful shift and rediscovery that can turn your life upside down and help you to work on the life path and goals you are actually wishing for, rather than living the life you thought you had to for whatever reasons. Using your intuition to guide you along the way can help, but it won't always be accessible and here's why: when you are in an awakening experience, you are dealing with your past and your present problems so that you can invest in a greater future.

Your processing experience is what will have to happen in order for you to be able to live in value to your chakra energies. What this means is that you will have to enjoy the turmoil of poking your internal hornet's nest, so to speak. Whatever you are going through right now, today has likely had a connection to the energy of your past that has been locked into your 7 chakras. In order to find your way into a new balance, you will have to see, know, feel and sense things that might have caused you pain in the past that are presently manifesting as other issues, like chronic pain, chronic fatigue syndrome, hormone imbalances, depression or anxiety, and so on.

There are ways that you can help yourself have a smoother, lighter, and more carefree and joyful journey as you stimulate the negative energies that you are working to let go of and purge. Troubleshooting chakra awakening is a part of the process that will help you to stay grounded and putting your best intentions and focus on healing.

The following list provides you with some key points about what you should avoid or be aware of as you go through the purging and cleansing experience.

- Avoid processed foods, as well as high sugar content foods and drinks, alcohol, and drugs. All of these chemicals have a powerful interaction with your energy and your vital organ systems. If you actually want to heal your chakras and your whole body, then you may have to make some significant changes in your diet and nutrition.

- Avoid attitudes and behaviors that will perpetuate bad habits and negativity. Seek to have a more positive outlook and be open to letting go of patterns that cause you to feel unhealthy.

- Avoid situations, people and environments that feel 'toxic' to you. There are a lot of scenarios that are unhealthy for people and sometimes we just go along with it because we feel like we have to. Part of stimulating a healing process and purging the negativity in our bodies is the letting go of particular people, places or activities that keep us feeling 'off' in our world.

- Avoid participating in anything that causes you physical or emotional harm or pain. Some events in life are unavoidable and we cannot control everything, but we can control some things and if you are repeatedly offering yourself something painful, it will cost your healing journey and cause it to take a lot longer.

- Avoid extremes. Extremes could be anything like binge-watching television for several days in a row, to drinking to excess, to uprooting and changing your job or living situation out of nowhere. These things may be tempting and are often coping mechanisms when we are uncomfortable with our awakening experiences. Looking for healthier ways to process is a much better action for the chakras.

- Process your opening with a healthy diet, sleep practice, hydration, and quality of life that will feel supportive and compatible with how you are going through your chakra awakening.

- Explore alternative methods for health care, like yoga, acupuncture, Reiki, massage, lymphatic drainage, sound baths, and deprivation tanks. All of these methods are ways that you can connect more deeply to the process of helping your chakra energy shift and heal. Self-care is a huge problem in our culture; most people have not learned how to make it a regular part of everyday life.

- Arrange for space to be alone and have quiet, reflective moments. It doesn't have to be a meditation or a specific practice; it can simply be having solitude and journaling or contemplating what your present feelings or state of mind is.

- Develop daily routines and habits that support your chakra awakening and healing journey. You don't have to do everything all at once; that would be too extreme. Start slowly and change one thing at a time to include more healthy energy healing practices.

- Be patient and kind to yourself. This awakening experience is about you and your life and how you want to live well. It can be easy to go overboard and feel unhappy with your progress, or like you aren't doing enough. That kind of belief or attitude will just cause even more negative energy for you to release, purge and heal, and so it is best to help yourself feel well along the journey.

All of these types of things can take time to find balance with and incorporate into a new lifestyle and routine. It's never easy to just change everything all at once and that is why it is best to plan for a long road to travel and that as you slowly start making some changes your chakras will start to change with you.

One of the biggest issues that we all have in our modern

age is instant gratification. Everyone wants a miracle cure, or easy fix to a lot of problems or life issues and the number one way that people fall off the chakra awakening wagon is to give up and stay with their lower vibrational energy because it is easy, familiar, and it doesn't require any hard work.

Awakening your chakras isn't hard, especially if you are wanting to create a more balanced and healthy life. It can actually be a joyful and pleasurable experience for a person to experience and as long as you have that attitude about it going in, you are likely to have a much better time hanging in there when things feel a little rough around the edges.

One major aspect of this practice is that you will have to go over it on a daily or regular basis in order to make the really big, positive changes and shifts. If you are not ready to make that a part of your life habits, then you may need more time to do some research and mentally prepare for the possibilities of making so much change in your life.

So, here are some additional tips to help you stay focused and avoid issues that may come up along the road:

- Make time for you.

- Make time for healing work, such as meditation, yoga, Reiki, etc.

- Help yourself by changing what isn't good for you (food, alcohol, lack of exercise).

- Practice daily, or regularly.

- Have patience and compassion for yourself.

- Pay attention to your intuition and let it help you make wise decisions about your healing path.

- Let go of the things in your life that are causing you pain, harm, or misfortune.

- Demand space for your growth and awakening.

- Get plenty of good rest and sleep.

- Keep yourself hydrated.

- Accept that change is inevitable and that nothing is permanent.

You can really help yourself open a lot more quickly and pleasantly when you are practicing healthy choices and working with your intuition as you go. There are certainly times where we will not have space for these exercises or energy clearing methods and that's okay. Life is full of ups and downs, ebbs and flows. There will be plenty of opportunities throughout your chakra awakening experience when you will need to just go with the flow.

- Avoid being rigid and overbearing with your healing experience.

- Avoid engineering impossible goals pertaining to your energy awakening.

- Avoid criticizing your lack of movement forward, especially if you need to just hold space for an important part of your healing work and give time to resettle and transform your energy.

- Avoid living in doubt or fear that you won't be able to do this work and just let it come forward in the right moments for you.

- Avoid boxing yourself into only one way of going through chakra awakening. The experience will be unique to you, so trust your intuition.

Anything that comes up along the way is likely meant to help you resolve some of the physical, mental, and emotional issues that have been a part of your blocked chakra system. It is absolutely normal for there to be strong feelings and emotions surfacing along the way. It is also partly true that things might get a little worse before they start to feel better.

When you are releasing serious illness, trauma, and old wounds from years ago, it can take some time to process and release; but, don't worry! As long as you are taking good care of yourself, trusting your intuition, avoiding things that will set you back, and making space for healing, you will be in good standing and the process will go that much more quickly for you.

Engage with the positive ways you can manage and maintain your chakra awakening experience and prepare to be amazed at how exciting it is to transform through healing your chakras.

You will read through each chakra again, from the root to the crown, to understand each one's imbalances within these categories of self-expression.

Chapter 27. Conclusion

Congratulations on finishing the book! If you have read through the entire book, then you are now equipped with the basic knowledge necessary to balance your chakras, free yourself from toxic energy, and experience real healing.

If you are skipping around the book, that's fine too. This book isn't a novel that you are supposed to read once and put aside, it's more like a manual that you should keep on hand so that you know how to deal with any issue that may arise. Reading through the information in this book once is helpful, but you'll need to meditate on the deeper meaning and take concrete steps if you truly want to own this wisdom.

It's all part of the spiritual journey that every one of us is on, whether we know it or not. This book has only scratched the surface of the great mountain of wisdom that has been stored up by countless generations of spiritual seekers.

Now, you are a part of this great chain of humanity that stretches back into the mists of ancient history. Your spiritual potential is unlimited, the only question is how far you are willing to go.

Radiating Energy

The road ahead of you might be long, but if you are open to the universe you will never run out of energy. We live in a universe made of energy. It flows into us and we radiate it out. One of the reasons that we were put on this earth is to play our part in the infinite chain of energy exchange that connects all life and matter in this universe.

It's all about perspective. People without this wide view are often held back from fully embracing practices like yoga and meditation. It is the idea that these are self-centered activities. The thought of spending extended periods of time looking inward can feel like a luxury or an indulgence when the outside world seems to demand our attention at all hours of the day. But the reality is that this whole idea is completely backward. People who are able to look inside of themselves and achieve personal balance are in the best position to bring healing to the entire world.

If you have ever flown on an airplane, then you've seen the song and dance where an airline representative tells you that in case of an emergency, you need to put your own oxygen mask on before you help anyone else. This can seem cruel at first, but it actually speaks to a deep truth. So many people try and sacrifice their own well-being to protect others, only to end up dragging everyone down in the process. If you try to put an oxygen mask on your child, then both of you are likely to end up unconscious. If you try to raise the energy of the world around you without balancing your own energies, then you're just as likely to bring the energy down.

Taking the time to balance your energies and raise your vibration doesn't need to take an eternity. Spending a few minutes, a day in yoga and meditation can create a recognizable uptick in energy. And this energy can be contagious. That's because this world isn't a zero-sum game, where everyone is fighting over a set amount of energy. The truth is that just as each chakra is part of a larger system, the same goes for each person. As each of us balance our own energies, the overall flow of energy increases and the vibration of the species is raised.

One thing you will learn as you discover the deep truths that exist within you and around you is that it's all the same. The systems that exist within you also exist within the planet. The only difference is the scale.

That's the beautiful message of all of this, everything is connected. By healing yourself, you are working to heal the planet. This doesn't mean that you need to feel responsible for the entire world, but it does mean that you don't need to feel like you are helpless in the face of a cold and uncaring world. The truth is that you're a part of a world that is alive and vibrating with the energy of billions of souls.

Today is your chance to heal yourself and heal the world. We're a long way from perfect, but it's like they say, the first step is always the hardest.

www.ingramcontent.com/pod-product-compliance
Lightning Source LLC
Chambersburg PA
CBHW070652250726
48662CB00001B/89